DR. COLBERT'S GUIDE to VITAMINS & SUPPLEMENTS

DON COLBERT, MD

SILOAM

Most Charisma House Book Group products are available at special quantity discounts for bulk purchase for sales promotions, premiums, fund-raising, and educational needs. For details, write Charisma House Book Group, 600 Rinehart Road, Lake Mary, Florida 32746, or telephone (407) 333-0600.

Dr. Colbert's Guide to Vitamins and Supplements
by Don Colbert, MD
Published by Siloam
Charisma Media/Charisma House Book Group
600 Rinehart Road
Lake Mary, Florida 32746
www.charismahouse.com

Cover design by Lisa Rae McClure
Design Director: Justin Evans

Visit the author's website at DrColbert.com.

Library of Congress Cataloging-in-Publication Data:
Names: Colbert, Don, author.
Title: Dr. Colbert's guide to vitamins and supplements : be empowered to make well-informed decisions / Don Colbert, MD
Other titles: Guide to vitamins and supplements
Description: Lake Mary, Florida : Siloam, [2016]
Identifiers: LCCN 2016045385| ISBN 9781629987637 (paperback) | ISBN 9781629987644 (ebook)
Subjects: LCSH: Dietary supplements--Therapeutic use. | Vitamin therapy. | BISAC: HEALTH & FITNESS / Vitamins.
Classification: LCC RM235.5 .C65 2016 | DDC 615.8/54--dc23
LC record available at https://lccn.loc.gov/2016045385

This book contains the opinions and ideas of its author. It is solely for informational and educational purposes and should not be regarded as a

Portions of this book were previously published by Siloam as *The Seven Pillars of Health,* ISBN 978-1-59979-094-7, copyright © 2013; *Reversing Diabetes,* ISBN 978-1-61638-598-9, copyright © 2012; *Dr. Colbert's "I Can Do This" Diet,* ISBN 978-1-61638-2674, copyright © 2011; *Eat This and Live for Kids,* ISBN 978-1-61638-1387, copyright © 2010; *Fasting Made Easy,* ISBN 978-1-59185-4517, copyright © 2004; *Get Fit and Live!,* ISBN 978-1-61638-0267, copyright © 2010; *Get Healthy Through Detox and Fasting,* ISBN 978-1-59185-9611, copyright © 2006; *Living in Divine Health,* ISBN 978-1-59185-8850, copyright © 2005; *The Rapid Waist Reduction Diet,* ISBN 978-1-62136-0445, copyright © 2013; *Stress Less,* ISBN 978-1-59979-3139, copyright © 2008; *Toxic Relief* (Revised & Expanded), ISBN 978-1-61638-5996, copyright © 2012; *What You Don't Know May Be Killing You,* ISBN 978-1-59185-2179, copyright © 2003; *The Bible Cure for ADD and Hyperactivity,* ISBN 978-0-88419-7447, copyright © 2001; *The Bible Cure for Allergies,* ISBN 978-0-88419-6853, copyright © 2000; *The Bible Cure for Arthritis,* ISBN 978-0-88419-6495, copyright © 1999; *The Bible Cure for Asthma,* 978-1-59185-2827, copyright © 2004; *The Bible Cure for Autoimmune Diseases,* ISBN 978-0-88419-9397, copyright © 2004; The *Bible Cure for Back Pain,* ISBN 978-0-88419-8307, copyright © 2002; *The Bible Cure for Candida and Yeast Infections,* ISBN 978-0-88419-7430, copyright © 2001; *The Bible Cure for High Cholesterol,* ISBN 978-1-59185-2414, copyright © 2004; *The Bible Cure for Colds and Flu,* ISBN 978-0-88419-9380, copyright © 2004; *The Bible Cure for Headaches,* ISBN 978-0-88419-6822, copyright © 2000; *The Bible Cure for Heartburn,* ISBN 978-0-88419-6518, copyright © 1999; *The Bible Cure for Hepatitis and Hepatitis C,* ISBN 978-0-88419-8291, copyright © 2002; *The*

Bible Cure for Irritable Bowel Syndrome, ISBN 978-0-88419-8277, copyright © 2002; *The Bible Cure for Memory Loss,* ISBN 978-0-88419-7461, copyright © 2001; *The Bible Cure for Menopause,* ISBN 978-0-88419-6839, copyright © 2000; *The Bible Cure for PMS and Mood Swings,* ISBN 978-0-88419-7454, copyright © 2001; *The Bible Cure for Prostate Disorders,* ISBN 978-0-88419-8284, copyright © 2002; *The Bible Cure for Skin Disorders,* ISBN 978-0-88419-8314, copyright © 2002; *The Bible Cure for Thyroid Disorders,* ISBN 978-1-59185-2810, copyright © 2004; *The Bible Cure Recipes for Overcoming Candida,* ISBN 978-0-88419-9403, copyright © 2004; *The New Bible Cure for Cancer,* ISBN 978-1-59979-8660, copyright © 2010; *The New Bible Cure for Chronic Fatigue and Fibromyalgia,* ISBN 978-1-59979-8677, copyright © 2011; *The New Bible Cure for Depression and Anxiety,* ISBN 978-1-59979-7601, copyright © 2009; *The New Bible Cure for Diabetes,* ISBN 978-1-59979-7595, copyright © 2009; *The New Bible Cure for Heart Disease,* ISBN 978-1-59979-8691, copyright © 2010; *The New Bible Cure for High Blood Pressure,* ISBN 978-1-61638-6153, copyright © 2013; *The New Bible Cure for Osteoporosis,* ISBN 978-1-59979-7571, copyright © 2009; *The New Bible Cure for Sleep Disorders,* ISBN 978-1-59979-7588, copyright © 2009; *The New Bible Cure for Stress,* ISBN 978-1-59979-8684, copyright © 2011; and *The New Bible Cure for Weight Loss,* ISBN 978-1-61638-6160, copyright © 2013.

16 17 18 19 20 — 9 8 7 6 5 4 3 2 1
Printed in the United States of America

CONTENTS

Part IV
An A-to-Z Guide

ABBREVIATIONS

25-hydroxyvitamin D3 (25-OHD3)
5-hydroxytryptophan (5-HTP)
5-lipoxygenase (5-LOX)
acetyl L-carnitine (ALC)
adenosine diphosphate (ADP)
adenosine triphosphate (ATP)
adequate intake (AI)
advanced glycation end products (AGEs)
alanine aminotransferase (ALT) test
alpha hydroxy acids (AHA)
alpha-linolenic acid (ALA)
Alpha-Tocopherol, Beta-Carotene Cancer Prevention (ATBC) trial
American Cancer Society (ACS)
amyotrophic lateral sclerosis (ALS)/ Lou Gehrig's disease
antigen leukocyte cellular antibody test (ALCAT)
attention deficit disorder (ADD)
attention-deficit hyperactivity disorder (ADHD)
basal metabolic rate (BMR)
benign prostatic hypertrophy (BPH)
body mass index (BMI)
carbon dioxide (CO_2)
Centers for Disease Control and Prevention (CDC)
chronic fatigue syndrome (CFS)
coenzyme Q_{10} (CoQ_{10})
congestive heart failure (CHF)
C-reactive protein (CRP)
cyclooxygenase-2 (COX-2)
daily reference value (DRV)
daily value (DV)
deglycyrrhizinated licorice (DGL)
dehydroepiandrosterone (DHEA)
Department of Health and Human Services (DHHS)
De-Stress Formula (DSF)
dichloro-diphenyl-trichloroethane (DDT)
diindolylmethane (DIM)
docosahexaenoic acid (DHA)
eicosapentaenoic acid (EPA)
Environmental Protection Agency (EPA)
Environmental Working Group (EWG)
eosinophilia-myalgia syndrome (EMS)
epigallocatechin gallate (EGCG)
ethylenediaminetetraacetic acid (EDTA)
fermentable oligosaccharides, disaccharides, monosaccharides, and polyols (FODMAP)
fructooligosaccharides (FOS)
gamma-aminobutyric acid (GABA)
gamma-linolenic acid (GLA)
gastrointestinal (GI)
glutathione (GSH)
gram(s) (g)
Gruppo Italiano per lo Studio della Streptochinasi nell'Infarto Miocardico (GISSI-Prevenzione)
Helicobacter pylori (H. pylori)
high-density lipoprotein (HDL)
hydrochloric acid (HCL)

Indole-3-Carbinol (I3C)
inorganic phosphate (Pi)
international units (IU)
irritable bowel syndrome (IBS)
low-density lipoprotein (LDL)
luteinizing hormone (LH)
magnetic resonance imaging (MRI)
methylenetetrahydrofolate reductase (MTHFR)
methylsulfonylmethane (MSM)
methyltetrahydrofolate (MTHF)
microgram(s) (mcg)
milligram(s) (mg)
milliliter(s) (ml)
millimeters of mercury (mmHg)
monosodium glutamate (MSG)
multiple sclerosis (MS)
N-acetyl cysteine (NAC)
NADH quinone oxidoreductase 1 (NQO1)
nanogram/milliliter (ng/ml)
National Center for Complementary and Integrative Health (NCCIH)
National Institutes of Health (NIH)
nicotinamide adenine dinucleotide hydrate (NADH)
nitric oxide (NO)
ounce(s) (oz.)
oxygen radical absorbance capacity (ORAC)
pentacyclic oxindole alkaloids (POAs)
perchloroethylene (perc, PCE)
phosphatidylserine (PS)
phosphatidylcholine (PC)
polychlorinated biphenyl (PCB)
polyethylene terephthalate (PETE)
PolyGlycopleX (PGX)
p-Phenylenediamine (PPD)
premature ventricular contraction (PVC)
premenstrual syndrome (PMS)
prisoner of war (POW)
prostaglandin 3 (PG3)
prostate-specific antigen (PSA)
pyrroloquinoline quinone (PQQ)
rapid eye movement (REM)
R-dihydrolipoic acid (R-DHLA)
reactive oxygen species (ROS)
recommended daily intake (RDI)
red blood cell (RBC)
ribonucleic acid (RNA)
S-adenosyl methionine (SAM-e)
selective serotonin reuptake inhibitors (SSRIs)
superoxide dismutase (SOD)
tablespoon (Tbsp.)
thyroid-stimulating hormone (TSH)
thyroxine (T4)
triiodothyronine (T3)
trimethylglycine (TMG)
upper limit (UL)
US Department of Agriculture (USDA)
US Pharmacopeia (USP)
World Health Organization (WHO)

PART I

THE EFFECTS OF OUR NUTRITIONAL LACK

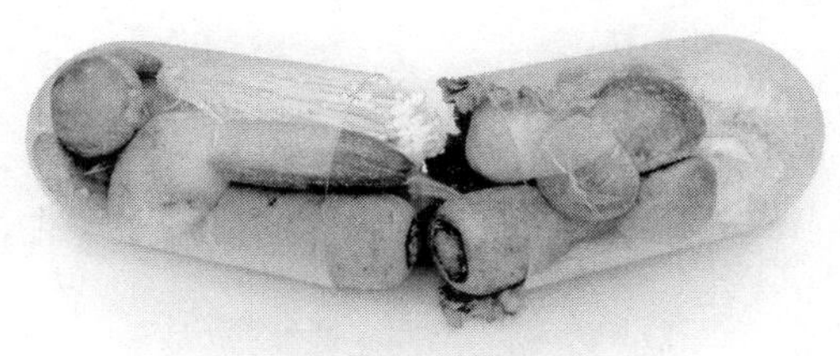

Chapter 1

YOUR NUTRITIONAL DEFICIT

WHILE MANY YEARS have passed since its publication, the study is still cited by medical authorities and referenced worldwide. I refer to the 2002 publication in the *Journal of the American Medical Association*—one of the leading medical journals in the United States—of research that recommended all adults take a multivitamin supplement to help prevent chronic diseases.[1] The findings shocked the medical community. During previous decades most of the medical establishment had insisted multivitamins were not necessary because people obtained all the vitamins and minerals they needed from their food. Some doctors theorized that multivitamins only gave people "expensive urine."

But the authors' findings went directly against this conventional wisdom and were based on hard data. Researchers reviewed studies of the relationships between vitamin intake and various diseases published between 1966 and 2002. They concluded that when people did not take in enough vitamins, they were at increased risk of a variety of chronic diseases, including heart disease and cancer. The best course, said the authors, was for all adults to take nutritional supplements.[2] While the study flabbergasted the medical community, the bias against multivitamins and supplements remains so strong that some doctors still won't recommend them. They insist that multivitamin supplements, and most other supplements, are "alternative therapy" or should only be recommended for sick and elderly patients who are more vulnerable to vitamin deficiencies. Unfortunately these doctors don't appreciate the extensiveness of vitamin deficiencies and the problems they create for people's health.

Most Common Nutritional Deficiencies[3]

- Vitamin D
- Vitamin K_2
- Calcium
- Iron (in women)
- Omega-3 Fats
- Magnesium
- Iodine
- Choline
- Vitamin E
- Vitamin A
- Vitamin B_{12} (in elderly)

WHY DIET ISN'T ENOUGH

In a perfect world the human body would indeed get all the nutrients it needs from food. The vitamins and minerals our bodies need to thrive *should* come through the foods we eat. However, processed foods have been stripped of much of their nutrient content. Cooking and storage are also reasons why our food loses more nutrients. Our toxic environment and toxins in our food, water, and air, coupled with our overstressed lifestyles, have increased our nutrient requirements. Even if we were to eat adequate fruits and vegetables, the nutrient content in them has decreased due to our depleted soils.

Few—if any—people get the nutrients they need from food alone, even if they eat a healthy diet. That's why a cornerstone of good health is nutritional supplements, since they will give you the nutrients you are likely missing from your normal diet. Those nutrients are the building blocks of health, and they will protect you against disease. Without them you are likely to have nutrient deficiencies.

It's extremely difficult to get all the nutrition your body needs from diet alone. Admittedly I do have very few patients who are incredibly meticulous about their diets. They pay attention to everything they eat, keeping diet logs to monitor what they will eat and when. Some are vegetarians; many insist on eating only raw foods (fruits, veggies, nuts, and seeds) or foods made and prepared according to healthy standards. They end up spending much of their time planning what to eat, shopping for food, and preparing their food. For a few, the time and energy it takes to plan can consume their lives.

God's Cure for Depleted Soil

In biblical times God told His people to work the land for six years and during the seventh year to give the land a "Sabbath rest" (Lev. 25:1–7). In so doing, the soil had time to regenerate its nutrients.

As I have mentioned, a major reason diet alone is not enough is because today's soil has fewer nutrients in it than ever before. When soil has fewer nutrients, so do the things that grow in it. Today's soil has suffered massively at the hands of agribusiness giants that plant and harvest produce on a large scale, aiming not for nutritious crops, but for crops that look good and last a long time on store shelves. Unfortunately nutrition has been sacrificed along the way. Long gone are the days when farmers rotated crops or mulched their fields, all of which preserved minerals in the soil. Now agribusinesses overwork the fields and add back a narrow range of minerals instead of letting the land naturally regenerate its nutrients.

According to the 1992 Earth Summit, North America has the worst soil in the world—85 percent of vital minerals have been depleted from it.[4] People noticed this trend as far back as 1936, when the U.S. Senate issued Document 264, which said that impoverished soil in the United States no longer provided plant foods with minerals needed for human nourishment.[5]

Today modern farmers fertilize the soil with a limited number of nutrients—mainly nitrogen, phosphorus, and potassium. These three nutrients have been found to grow big, beautiful crops, but they are only a few of the dozens our bodies need to be healthy. Shiny apples or deep green lettuce bunches on grocery store shelves may look beautiful, but the beauty is only skin deep. They are usually poor in many nutrients because they were grown in depleted soil.

Many studies show how depleted soil has affected the mineral content of vegetables and fruits. One observer compared the data from the US Department of Agriculture (USDA) handbook from 1972 to the USDA food tables of today and found dramatic reductions in nutrient content. For example, nearly half the calcium and vitamin A in broccoli have disappeared. The vitamin A content in collard greens has fallen to nearly half its previous levels. Potassium dropped from 400 mg to 170 mg, and magnesium fell from 57 mg to only 9 mg. Cauliflower lost almost half of its vitamin C, thiamine, and riboflavin. The calcium in pineapple went from 17 mg to 7 mg. Those astonishing losses in nutrients eventually will have a significant impact on your health.[6]

Acid rain is another culprit in soil degradation. Even a modest amount of acid rain causes soil to lose nutrients. One thirty-year study showed that acid rain steadily depleted the soils of the forest by 38 percent at one site in South Carolina and made the soil more acidic.[7] Another that examined nutritional data for the second half of the twentieth century revealed declines in the amount of protein, calcium, phosphorus, iron, and various vitamins for forty-three different vegetables and fruits.[8] I believe the depletion of our soil is part of the curse God placed on the land after Adam and Eve were forced to leave the Garden of Eden. But I also believe that as we come under God's grace, He has blessed us with the tools and the knowledge that will make our land—and our food—rich in nutrients again.

Good Grains—How They Rank

It's almost impossible to rank grains because we need to consider all the different elements involved (size, soil, and so on). Each grain is different, with its own texture and taste. Each also has different nutrients, including fiber, B vitamins, and trace minerals, that refined grain products do not contain. Barley, oats, millet, rye, quinoa, and brown rice are some of the healthiest grains.[9]

Poor Digestion

Another reason people need nutritional supplements is because of poor digestion. I will occasionally do a blood test to check intracellular nutrient levels for certain patients, and very often they are deficient in several nutrients, even if they eat a healthy diet and take supplements. This is because it's not just what you eat but also what you assimilate and absorb into your body.

An estimated one hundred million Americans have some type of digestive disorder.[10] This means that even if they put nutritious foods in their mouths, the nutrients may not be adequately absorbed by their bodies. One reason for poor digestion is lack of enzymes in the diet. Enzymes are essential to the body's digestion, assimilation, and absorption of food. But many adults do not have enough enzymes that are essential for normal digestion. This could be for a number of reasons:

1. They choose highly processed food that is void of enzymes.
2. They do not properly chew their food properly, making it difficult for enzymes to break down the food. Each bite should be chewed thirty times.
3. They cook food at high temperatures, destroying the enzymes in the food.
4. They consume excessive amounts of fluids with their meals, which washes out their enzymes and hydrochloric acid.

Also, as we grow older, our capacity to make enzymes diminishes. Stress also hinders digestive enzymes from being produced.

Quick Quiz

Most digestion takes place in the:

A. Stomach B. Small intestine C. Large intestine

Answer: B. Small intestine.

Many people, especially individuals over fifty years of age, have low levels of hydrochloric acid, which is needed for proper digestion. In addition, millions of Americans are consuming antacids and medications that block acid, such as Pepcid, Mylanta, Zantac 75, Prilosec, Nexium, and other medications that reduce hydrochloric acid. Other people have poor digestion because they are stressed or are on birth control pills or other medications that affect how well vitamins are absorbed. Each of these may contribute to vitamin and mineral deficiencies. Also almost every medication causes a loss of vitamins, minerals, or antioxidants.

The bottom line is that to be healthy you almost certainly need to start taking nutritional supplements. Consult your physician before beginning any supplements. I will review which ones to take, and in what quantities, in part 2. In the remainder of part 1, though, I will review what the lack of nutrients is doing to us, such as the toxins we face (including stress), and how metabolism affects weight.

Chapter 2

WHAT'S IN YOUR FOOD AND WATER

IMAGINE YOU HAVE two shelves in your pantry, one labeled "Dead Food" and the other, "Living Food." On the dead shelf the tag reads: "These foods will make you disease-prone; will cause degenerative diseases, such as diabetes, cardiovascular disease, and arthritis; and will make you obese. They will also make you fatigued and prone to develop hypertension and high cholesterol." But the tag on the living shelf says: "These foods will protect your body from cancer, heart disease, Alzheimer's disease, all degenerative diseases, and obesity, and they will sharpen your mind, energize you, and enliven you."

This stark, but realistic, choice faces everyone. As an average American, you may be consuming up to five pounds of food each day.[1] Over your lifetime that means approximately seventy tons of food will pass through your intestinal tract and be assimilated by your body.

Living Longer—But Better?

Life expectancy in the United States increased to 78.8 years in 2012, according to a report from the Centers for Disease Control and Prevention. The question is, what is the quality of this longer life? About seventy million adults have high blood pressure, nearly one in every three. More than one-third are obese. Both conditions leave people feeling sluggish and unhealthy.[2] Alzheimer's disease is projected to nearly triple by 2050.[3]

Which shelf are you going to select food from? Remember, they are not imaginary; in your pantry, freezer, and fridge right now are foods that lead to life—or death. They are probably all mixed together. Processed peanut butter sits next to extra-virgin olive oil, and oatmeal, next to an XXL-size bag of potato chips.

To help you better grasp the need for vitamins and supplements, you need to understand how the food you eat affects your health, and why today's food doesn't contain all the nourishment you need. This truth can be exacerbated when you fail to consume living foods, which contribute to good health. Everything you put in your mouth has the potential to produce life or death. While food is a reward that can bring blessings, eating the wrong foods can produce curses of poor health.

"Why Does It Matter What I Eat?"

All foods are *not* created equal. In fact, some food should not be labeled "food" but rather "consumable product" or "edible, but void of nourishment" or "dangerous to your health."

God created living foods for our consumption. They exist in a raw or close-to-raw state. Fruits, vegetables, grains, seeds, and nuts are beautifully packaged in divinely created wrappers called skins and peels. Living food looks robust, healthy, and alive. No chemicals have been added. It has not been bleached or chemically altered. It is plucked, harvested, and squeezed, not processed, packaged, and put on a shelf. Living foods are *recognizable* as food.

Dr. Colbert's List of Worst Fats to Consume

- Hydrogenated and partially hydrogenated fats and trans fats
- Excessive saturated fats
- Excessive polyunsaturated fats
- Deep fried fats

Dead foods are the opposite. They are living foods that have fallen into human hands and been altered in every imaginable way, making them last as long as possible at room temperature. Manufacturers make them as addictive as possible to the consumer. They add considerable amounts of sugar, which is usually called "dextrose," "corn syrup," "fructose," "glucose," and anything else ending in "-ose." They also create man-made fats that involve taking various oils and heating them to dangerously high temperatures so that the nutrients die. They get reborn as something completely different: a deadly, sludgy, toxic inflammatory substance. This sludge—called "hydrogenated" or "partially hydrogenated" oil—is a common ingredient in the American diet and is present in most processed foods.

Dead foods hit our bodies like a foreign intruder. Chemicals, including preservatives, food additives, and bleaching agents, place a strain on the liver. Toxic man-made fats form in our cell membranes and become incorporated in our bodies or stored as fats. They begin to form plaque in our arteries.

"FRANKEN-FOODS"

Why am I so opposed to man-made foods, whether fast food or processed food? Not only are they loaded with sodium; they also contain excessive sugars and toxic fats (you might call them "The Big 3"). These foods are the real killers in the standard American diet.

I like to call the processed foods that help fatten up so many people "Franken-foods." They are a nightmare and a primary reason you should limit your intake of processed foods, such as white bread, instant white rice, crackers, chips, and sugary sweet treats. If processing food made it healthier, I would be its biggest advocate. However, without exception it is higher in depleted flours, sugar, salt, food additives, and usually toxic fats. The process that produces these dangerous foods strips away valuable vitamins, minerals, fiber, enzymes, phytonutrients, and antioxidants. Most processed foods have a high glycemic index and raise your blood sugar, causing weight gain and inflammation and setting the stage for most degenerative diseases.

With dead, processed food you get the worst and lose the best. And yet food companies hire the brightest minds and chemists to make their foods as addictive as possible, so you can't eat just a little bit. They know how to create the eye appeal, tastes, textures, feels, and smells people find irresistible.

It is high time for you to boot the following dead foods out of your life. This next section lists some primary culprits that you need to eliminate or drastically reduce.

THE BAD AND THE UGLY

Monosodium glutamate (MSG)

A common ingredient in processed foods, and one of the most dangerous and best disguised, is MSG. MSG is the sodium salt of an amino acid—glutamic acid—and looks similar to sugar or salt. MSG doesn't alter the taste of food the way salt and other seasonings do. Instead it "enhances" taste by increasing the sensitivity of your taste buds. In other words, it tricks your brain into thinking the food tastes good. Many food manufacturers add MSG to stimulate your appetite and get you to become addicted to their products. Researchers have found that giving rats MSG increased their food intake by 40 percent.[4]

Adverse Reactions

Generally the more salty or processed a food is, the more MSG, or "free glutamate," the food contains.

Glutamate, or glutamic acid, comes in a bound form and a free form. Both are found in natural protein-rich foods, such as most meats, most dairy products, seaweed, mushrooms, tomatoes, fermented soy products, yeast extracts, hydrolyzed proteins, nuts, and legumes.

Only the "free" form can enhance the food's flavor. Free glutamic acid is metabolized to MSG in the body. Most of our MSG intake is found in processed foods, such as soups, gravies, salad dressings, soy sauce, Worcestershire sauce, processed meats, and frozen entrees. It is found in most crackers, potato chips, and corn chips. It is hidden not only in most store-bought processed foods, but also in many of the processed foods—such as fried chicken products, sausage, scrambled egg mix, and grilled chicken fillets—at restaurants, including Chick-fil-A and KFC.

Research confirms that MSG consumed by lab animals causes brain lesions of the hypothalamus. Neuroscientists generally agree that glutamic acid (present in MSG) is neurotoxic and kills neurons by exciting them to death. MSG may damage the hypothalamus, which controls appetite. A damaged hypothalamus can lead to a runaway appetite. MSG also causes the pancreas to produce more insulin. The blood sugar often drops due to the excessive insulin and typically makes you hungry. That's why many people are hungry an hour or so after eating food containing MSG. MSG also blocks the message to the brain that you are full or satisfied and interferes with appetite hormones.

High-sugar foods and beverages

Refined sugar is a man-made product, unlike the natural sugars with fiber found in living food. Why is processed sugar so harmful? Because it is inflammatory and it can make you fat. When you overeat sugar, your body goes into fat-storage mode by raising insulin levels. That's why most diabetics gain weight when they begin taking insulin—often as much as twenty or thirty pounds. Sugar creates a cycle of demand for more sugar, which raises insulin levels. Insulin is a powerful hormone that signals the body to store fat.

To Diet or Not to Diet Soda?

Many people think diet sodas help them lose weight, but one study showed otherwise. A study covering eight years of collected data showed that your risk of becoming overweight by drinking one to two cans of soda per day is 32.8 percent, but your risk increases to 54.5 percent if you drink one to two cans of diet soda instead.[5]

In addition, sugar impairs your immune system, temporarily impairs the T-cells that protect you against viruses, and also temporarily impairs the B-cells, which produce antibodies.

It impairs white blood cells called phagocytes, which protect you from bacteria. Sugar also feeds cancer cells and is linked to behavioral disorders; there is a strong link between excessive sugar intake and attention deficit/hyperactivity disorder (ADHD).

Sugar leads to osteoporosis by creating an acidic environment in your tissues, which causes your body to cannibalize your bones. If you don't get enough calcium in your diet, your body may pull it from your bones and teeth to rebalance your pH, and you may develop bone loss and eventually osteoporosis.

There's more: it aggravates yeast problems, leads to type 2 diabetes, elevates cholesterol, and accelerates the aging process.

White flour

White bread is a poor choice for food. When water is added to white bread, it forms a sticky paste that constipates your body. Some people say it's so sticky they can almost hang wallpaper with it! It delivers little nutrition (even with all those added vitamins and minerals they advertise on the package) and converts to sugar rapidly. This "enriched flour" is anything but an enriched product.

In short, white bread is another example of how a wonderful, God-given food gets mugged on the way to the grocery shelf. All bread starts out as whole grain. To make white bread, the manufacturer removes the outer shell of the grain with all its healthy fiber and B vitamins. Then the nutrition-packed wheat germ is extracted. Both the fiber and the wheat germ are actually *resold to health food stores*. Meanwhile the denuded white flour heads to the mainstream market to be made into white bread, buns, pastries, crackers, pasta, most cereals, and other products.

Fast food

The typical American consumes three hamburgers and four orders of fries per week. In 1970 Americans spent approximately $6 billion on fast food. By 2000 spending had risen to more than $110 billion.[6] That ranked spending on fast food higher than on personal computers, computer software, new cars, and higher education combined. This trend hasn't slowed, either. In March of 2015, for the first time ever, sales at restaurants and bars overtook spending at grocery stores.[7]

Fast food contains especially high amounts of trans fats, which I will describe later. Acrylamides are toxic chemicals formed by the combustion of oil and hydrocarbons. They are highly carcinogenic—particularly associated with colon cancer—and should be avoided. Acrylamides cause cellular

DNA to mutate. French fries are among the worst offenders when it comes to foods containing acrylamides.

Deadly meats. These meats are best to eat rarely and eat fiber afterward, such as one tablespoon of chia seeds, to bind toxins and speed up the transit through the GI tract. The list starts with livers and kidneys. Since these are filtering organs that filter toxins, many toxins reside in these organs. By all means, avoid them.

Cold cuts and packaged meats, such as bologna, salami, hot dogs, bacon, sausage, and processed ham, are usually high in saturated fats, which are associated with heart disease, and are always high in salt. They also contain lots of nitrites and nitrates—fancy names for ugly substances that may form cancer-causing chemicals called nitrosamines or n-nitroso compounds. These compounds are associated with cancer of the bladder, esophagus, stomach, brain, and oral cavity. Bacon, sausage, and hot dogs are also high in saturated fats and chemicals.

Fats

Fats add delicious taste and "mouth feel" to foods, but often at a dangerous price. There are fats that kill (trans or hydrogenated fats and partially hydrogenated fats), fats that kill in excess but heal in moderation (saturated and polyunsaturated fats), and fats that heal (omega-3 fats and monounsaturated fats).

The fats you should avoid are trans fatty acids, often called "trans fats," such as hydrogenated and partially hydrogenated fats. You need to limit your consumption of saturated and polyunsaturated fats. Saturated fat is found mostly in animal fats. It is solid at room temperature and significantly raises the low-density lipoprotein (LDL), or bad, cholesterol. Polyunsaturated fats are found in products such as mayonnaise, salad dressings, grape seed oil, safflower oil, sunflower oil, and corn oil.

Trans fats. This includes hydrogenated and partially hydrogenated fats. They originated more than a century ago; a German scientist patented the process of hydrogenation in 1902. This involves mixing the cheapest oils—soy, corn, cottonseed, and canola—with a metal catalyst, usually nickel. The oil is subjected to hydrogen gas in a high-pressure, high-temperature reactor to force hydrogen through it until it is saturated. Emulsifiers are added, and the oil is deodorized at high temperatures and steam cleaned. Margarine is an example of a product containing hydrogenated oils; it must be bleached to hide its gray color and then dyed and flavored to resemble butter.

Dangerous Fat

The more solid the hydrogenated fat, the more dangerous it is to your body.

Adding hydrogen atoms to liquid fats and oils makes these oils stay in solid form at room temperature. This means that they are much less likely to become rancid, which prolongs their shelf life. However, this process alters the chemical structure of the fat to an unnatural "trans fatty acid," which becomes an enemy of the heart by raising LDL, bad, cholesterol levels and lowering high-density lipoprotein (HDL), good, cholesterol levels. Trans fats have been found to be more harmful to your arteries than saturated fat and are implicated in heart disease and cancer.

These bad fats are found in almost every item in the middle of a grocery store—where all the shelf-stable pastries, rolls, breakfast cereals, breakfast bars, crackers, and processed or packaged foods reside. Bad fats are also found in the bakery section in the doughnuts, pastries, cookies, cakes, pies, and other items.

Saturated fats. These fats are usually found in animal products but rarely in fruits and vegetables. Foods high in saturated fats include most selections at fast-food restaurants (i.e., hamburgers, fried chicken strips), dairy products, and commercial fried foods and processed foods, such as cookies, cakes, doughnuts, pies, and pastries.

Fatty Drippings

Meat drippings, such as beef tallow/dripping, lard (pork), chicken, duck, goose, bacon fat, and even turkey, contain a whopping 44.8 gm of saturated fat per 3.5-ounce serving. So the next time you cook those green beans, think twice about slathering them with bacon fat![8]

Saturated fats are also found in cured meats, such as bacon, sausage, ham, hot dogs, cold cuts, bologna, salami, and pepperoni. Red meats, duck, and goose meat are also usually quite high in saturated fats. Some vegetable oils, such as coconut oil, palm kernel oil, and palm oil, are also high in saturated fats.

I recommend limited intake of these fats rather than avoiding them because—in moderation—they provide benefits to the body. Saturated fats enhance our immune system and allow calcium to be incorporated into our bones. *In moderation* means no more than 6 percent of your total daily caloric intake should come from saturated fats.[9] Moderate amounts of saturated fats also protect the liver from toxins, help prevent breast cancer and colon cancer, and help promote weight loss. Coconut oil is my favorite saturated fat.

Polyunsaturated fats (omega-6 fats). Polyunsaturated fats oxidize much faster than monounsaturated fats. That is why these fats become rancid so quickly. Polyunsaturated fats are liquid at room temperature, while refrigerated, and when frozen. There are two families of polyunsaturated fats: the omega-3 fats and the omega-6 fats.

When polyunsaturated oils, such as corn oil, safflower oil, sunflower oil, sesame oil, soybean oil, cottonseed oil, grape seed oil, commercial salad dressings, and others, are used in cooking, and especially deep frying, oxidation occurs even faster. Oxidation also occurs in your arteries as free radicals attack the polyunsaturated fats, which are carried in LDL cholesterol.

Oxidized cholesterol is much more likely to form plaque in an artery or on arterial walls. As fats are broken down through oxidation, they form substances that promote blood clotting and cause inflammation—all of which make blood flow more difficult.

Polyunsaturated fats are not the worst fats, but they aren't the best, either. They come from healthy sources, but may tend to be overprocessed or oxidezed by the heating process by the time they reach the consumer. Eating too much polyunsaturated fat increases inflammation, which is associated with heart disease, arthritis, cancer, and Alzheimer's disease. However, polyunsaturated fats are essential for life and must be consumed daily in small amounts. The best way is with small portions of pecans, almonds, Brazil nuts, pine nuts, pistachios, and walnuts. If you must use vegetable oil, choose very small amounts of *cold-pressed* polyunsaturated fats (corn oil, flaxseed oil, hemp oil, pumpkinseed oil, safflower oil, grape seed oil, sesame oil, soybean oil, and sunflower oil) and do not cook with them. You can find these at most health food stores.

Precious Water

Water is the single most important nutrient for our bodies. It is involved in every function of our bodies. You can live five to seven weeks without food, but the average adult can last only about five to seven days without water.[10]

Despite its essential, life-giving qualities, many people never drink water. As a result, they live in a mildly dehydrated state with various irritating symptoms and never realize it. Some don't like the taste of water, or they were never taught the importance of drinking it. Maybe their parents gave them juice, soft drinks, milk—anything but water. As a result, many people spend their day going from one caffeinated or sugar-based drink to another. Little do they know that all that caffeine and sugar are actually stealing water from their bodies, doing them more harm than good.

H_2O 101

Two to three cups of water is lost a day just through perspiration through normal activity levels. At higher levels of activity people can sweat out about a quart of water. Your body also loses water daily through urination, elimination, and exhalation.[11]

In my practice, I see people all the time whose bodies are starved for clean, natural water. They are neglecting the most basic pillar of health, and their bodies and minds pay a terrible price. By the time I see them, they often suffer from headaches, back pain, arthritis, skin problems, digestion problems, and other ailments. Often they have seen another doctor, who might have given them medications that didn't address the problem but only turned off the symptoms. This is similar to a red warning light blinking on your car's dashboard, informing you to check your engine. If you simply decide to remove the fuse to turn off the warning light instead of taking your car in for service, you eventually will ruin your car's engine. The same is true of your body.

Take a Guess

What percentage of water does the average adult male's body contain?

A. 40–50 percent B. 50–60 percent C. 62–65 percent

Answer: C. The average adult male's body is 62 to 65 percent water, compared with women, whose bodies are 51 to 55 percent water. Men have more water in their bodies because they generally have more muscle mass, whereas women have a higher percentage of body fat.[12]

My wife, Mary, and I have lost count of the people who come up to us at seminars and say, "I had this or that problem, but I took your advice and started drinking water, and it went away." People tend to lose excess weight, their arthritis problems disappear, and their high blood pressure begins to return to normal levels. If it sounds like a miracle cure, that's because it is! God created us to rely on water for our very lives.

HARMFUL WATER

Now that I've (hopefully) convinced you of the necessity of water, I must add: all water is not created equal. While we should drink healthy amounts of water, we need to drink the right kind of water. Tap water is not it. I wish I could tell you that all water is the same, wherever it comes from, and that our body naturally filters out any "bad stuff." Not true. When there are harmful substances in our water, those substances get into our bodies. For more information, please refer to *The Seven Pillars of Health*.

While your body needs water, tap water may not be the best source. I am strongly convinced that over time it will diminish your quality of life. Even if you can't afford a two-hundred-dollar filtration system, you can begin by purchasing an inexpensive pitcher filtration system or a faucet-mounted filtration system, such as the ones manufactured by ZeroWater or a Seychelle alkaline water pitcher. You can find a solution within your financial means. Tap water is good for watering lawns, washing clothes, and flushing toilets, but not for drinking.

Chapter 3

UNEXPECTED SOURCES OF TOXINS

We are being bombarded with toxins daily. While you may not be aware of it, toxins enter our bodies through the air we breathe, the food we eat, the water we drink, and direct contact with our skin. In addition, there are some surprising sources of toxins you need to pay attention to.

Common Toxins

Here are some primary avenues by which toxins get into our bodies.

Air pollution

Much of the planet's air is unavoidably dirty. In major metropolitan cities—and even smaller areas with chemical plants and other industrial facilities—smog is so common that people hardly notice it anymore. In rural America pesticides, dust, and ozone contribute to the problem. Carbon monoxide from buses, cars, and airplanes; heavy metals and chemicals from factories and refineries; and smoke from agricultural and forest fires all contribute to the gaseous soup we breathe.

Indoor problems

Sometimes indoor air can be just as bad as outdoor air—and is usually worse. Chemicals, bacteria, mold, and mold toxins get trapped and recirculated throughout heating and air-conditioning systems of buildings. So do chemical compounds used in construction. New carpets and pressed wood release formaldehyde into your breathing air. Paints release unhealthy solvents. Water-damaged dry wall and ceiling tiles emit mold toxins.

Cigarette smoke is a major airborne health hazard in many homes. Even though many municipalities and states have banned smoking in public facilities, millions of people still smoke outdoors (ever pass by a hospital's exterior "smoking zone"?). According to the American Cancer Society (ACS), about half of all Americans who continue to smoke will die because of the habit. The ACS calls cigarette smoking the most significant risk for lung cancer and expected more than 221,000 new cases of this type of cancer (of more than 1.6 million overall) during 2015. Overall for that year the society forecast more than 589,000 cancer deaths.[1]

And the Winner Is...

Thirty percent of all cancer deaths are attributed to tobacco use, tying it with obesity as the number one risk factor associated with the disease.[2]

Food

Almost all nonorganically grown produce may be tainted by pesticides, herbicides, parasites, and chemicals. These toxins and microbes find their way into our food supply—and into our bodies.

Pesticides are absorbed in the intestinal tract from an animal's feed, and what is not detoxified by the animal's liver may be deposited in their fatty tissues. When you eat meat, pesticides and chemicals in the meat may eventually go into your fatty tissues—including the fatty tissues in your brain.

If you eat processed foods, you welcome a host of chemicals into your body, including synthetic dyes, flavoring agents, chemical preservatives, emulsifiers, texturizers, humectants, ripening gases, bleaching agents, and sugar substitutes, such as aspartame. Chemical food additives are usually made from—brace yourself—petroleum or coal tar products. Bleaching agents can be so toxic that Germany has banned their use in flour since 1958.[3]

Another common, but extremely dangerous, substance is pesticides. Some dangerous ones are banned in the United States but are still used by countries from which we import crops and foods. Those banned chemicals usually end up in our food supplies. Other toxic chemicals, such as dichloro-diphenyl-trichloroethane (DDT) and polychlorinated biphenyls (PCBs), have been banned in the United States for decades, but since these chemicals remain in our water, land, and air, fish and animal products continue to be main sources of DDT and PCBs in our diets. DDT was developed as a pesticide in the 1940s, and PCBs were first created and used as cooling fluids in the late 1920s. The Environmental Protection Agency (EPA) lists DDT and PCBs as probable human carcinogens since both cause liver cancer in laboratory animals.[4]

Parasites are another enemy of our food supply. One survey of public health laboratories reported that 15.6 percent of specimens examined contained a parasite.[5] Usually third world countries are major exporters of food to the United States. Often the conditions in which the food is handled and shipped to the States are less than sanitary, which leaves our food supply and, ultimately, our digestive systems vulnerable to parasites.[6] People who are eating more raw foods are predisposed to getting parasitic infections. Improper food handling and preparation also leave us exposed to intestinal parasites. Many times workers do not wash their hands before handling food that ends up on your plate.

AVOID HEAVY METAL

I don't mean heavy metal music. I mean such substances as mercury, cadmium, aluminum, and lead. Some people have so much metal in their bodies that they need chelation therapy—oral, intravenous, or suppository forms of chelation to remove metals from their bodies. One of my patients had amyotrophic lateral sclerosis (ALS), better known as Lou Gehrig's disease. Neurologists said she had only a few months to live. Barely able to walk into my office using a walker, she often had to use a wheelchair. After learning she had smoked heavily for forty years, I did a heavy metal screening of her and found off-the-charts amounts of cadmium in her urine. I started chelating this out of her body. She later returned to work full time. The neurologist later said he misdiagnosed her.

You should consume chlorophyll foods or supplement daily with supplements including wheat grass, barley grass, oat grass, healthy algae, and other supplements, to help detoxify from heavy metals. (For more information, please refer to my books *What You Don't Know May Be Killing You* and *Get Healthy Through Detox and Fasting.*[7])

Another source of toxins for millions of people is in their teeth. Amalgam fillings, which are also called silver fillings, are about 50 percent mercury and also usually contain tin, copper, and silver. About a million people every week receive amalgam fillings. The original fillings, made from 1850 until 1974, slowly released mercury over thirty years. However, since 1974, the fillings release enough mercury into the body to cause trouble within three to five years.[8] A typical filling contains 750,000 mcg of mercury and releases 10 mcg of mercury per day.[9]

When mercury enters the membrane of a cell, the body's immune system may identify it as an abnormal cell that must be destroyed. The immune system may then form antibodies against your body's normal cell because they appear abnormal since they contain mercury. This can lead to rheumatoid arthritis, Hashimoto's thyroiditis, Grave's disease, MS, lupus, and other autoimmune diseases. People suffering with heavy metal toxicity, as occurs in the slow release of mercury from amalgam fillings, usually don't notice right away because symptoms start slowly. The victims simply feel bad and say things such as, "I don't know what is wrong with me—I just don't feel good, and I am very tired."

For many years the dental community maintained that mercury was tightly bound with other metal components and did not escape from amalgam fillings. However, research has proved that mercury vapors do escape during chewing and brushing, and when contacted with hot or acidic food. One study found that levels of mercury vapor in the mouth after chewing were fifty-four times higher in people with amalgam fillings than in people without amalgams.[10] We now know it is physically impossible for mercury to be "locked in" the amalgam fillings once they are placed in the teeth.

The Agency for Toxic Substances and Disease Registry lists mercury as the third most toxic substance known to mankind[11]—more toxic than lead, cadmium, and arsenic. I'm amazed that dentists still put it into people's mouths. When a dentist removes a silver filling, he is required by the Occupational Safety and Health Administration to put the filling in a sealed biohazard container.

Down in the Mouth

If you have silver amalgam dental fillings, you eventually should consider having them removed, but be very careful about it. Many dentists have shared horror stories about patients who had their silver fillings removed and were in worse shape afterward.

There is a proper and safe way to have amalgam fillings removed. Begin by finding a willing and cooperative biological dentist who is aware of the risks of mercury and is knowledgeable about the proper way to remove silver amalgam fillings. He may use a controlled chewing test to determine the extent of mercury being released from your dental fillings. He may conduct electrical readings on your fillings to determine the sequence for removing fillings, perhaps removing the most negatively charged fillings first or fillings that are leaking first. To find a biological dentist, call the International College of Integrative Medicine (formerly Great Lakes College of Clinical Medicine) at (419) 303-9769, or visit its web site at www.icimed.com. Or, you can visit the site of the International Academy of Oral Medicine and Toxicology at www.iaomt.org. (Refer to my book *What You Don't Know May Be Killing You* for more information.)

And if the dentist recommends silver fillings for you or your children, learn the potential dangers of mercury, and refuse it. If he or she insists, then find another dentist. Porcelain crowns cost more up front, but it could save your health. Be aware that if you have composite fillings placed, they should be considered to be only temporary and should not be left in long term. Please do not run out and have all your silver fillings removed, or you may actually get sicker. Instead, find a good biological dentist who can safely and slowly remove them over a period of time.

Household Products

Solvents, which are used in cleaning products to dissolve materials that are not water soluble, contain toxins that, if they come into contact with your skin, are actually absorbed into your body. Remember, pharmaceutical companies are now using transdermal (through-the-skin) methods to deliver hormones, some blood pressure medicines, nicotine, and other drugs. If chemicals come in contact with the skin, realize that some of the chemical will be absorbed. In some cases most of the toxic chemical may be absorbed, especially certain solvents, cleaners, and so forth. Toxic household items include paint thinners, stain removers, varnishes, ammonia, bleach, glass cleaners, metal polish, and furniture polish.

Furniture and household items can emit toxins. For instance, formaldehyde, which is used in particleboard, carpet padding, carpet glues, upholstered furniture, curtains, and bedding, may cause fatigue and headaches. For example, petroleum distillates, found in metal polishes, can cause temporary eye clouding under short-term exposure. Longer exposure can damage the nervous system, skin, kidneys, and eyes.[12]

Phenol and cresol, found in disinfectants, are corrosive and can cause diarrhea, fainting, dizziness, and kidney and liver damage. Nitrobenzene, in furniture and floor polishes, can cause skin discoloration, shallow breathing, vomiting, and death, and is associated with cancer and birth defects.[13]

Don't Mix!

If you have ever mixed bleach and ammonia, you probably had an unpleasant surprise. Sodium hypochlorite, an ingredient of chlorine bleach, releases a toxic gas that if mixed with ammonia may cause mild asthmatic symptoms or more serious problems.[14]

Benzene is classified by the Environmental Working Group as a Class A carcinogen due to its link to an increased risk of leukemia. It is used in a wide range of products many of us encounter every day—carpet cleaners, cleaning fluids, conditioners, detergents, dyes, enamel sprays, furniture, gasoline, nail polishes, paint, paint removers, paint thinners, plastics, solvents, spot removers, spray acrylics, spray paints, stains/lacquers, vinyl floorings, wood finishes, wood lighteners, wood preservatives, and many other man-made products.[15]

In addition to household products, a study in 2006 raised questions about the benzene levels in some soft drinks, particularly those with orange, strawberry, pineapple, and cranberry flavors. Five percent of soft drinks studied had benzene levels that exceed the EPA limit for our drinking water. And buyers beware: even if a soft drink doesn't contain benzene when it is manufactured, if it contains vitamin C (ascorbic acid) and either sodium benzoate or potassium benzoate, benzene can form in it when it is exposed to heat and/or light.[16]

Perchloroethylene (also called perc, PCE, and tetrachloroethylene) and

1-1-1 trichloroethane solvents, found in spot removers and carpet cleaners, can cause liver and kidney damage if ingested. Perc, determined to be a carcinogen by the Department of Health and Human Services (DHHS), has caused liver and kidney tumors in laboratory animals.[17] Perc is commonly used in dry cleaning. To avoid adverse reactions from perc, be sure to remove the plastic wrapping from your dry-cleaned items and allow them to air out for several days before wearing or ironing them.

Switch to Natural Products

Most people may not realize that they have options. They don't have to purchase products containing harmful chemicals in order to clean their homes. Below are a couple natural products most people have in their pantries that can be used as household cleaners.

Lemon juice, which contains citric acid, is a deodorizer and can be used to clean glass and remove stains from aluminum, clothes, and porcelain. It is a mild lightener or bleach if used with sunlight.

Vinegar contains about 5 percent acetic acid, which makes it a mild acid. Because it is slightly acidic, vinegar is able to dissolve mineral deposits and grease, remove traces of soap, remove mildew or wax buildup, polish some metals, and deodorize. Vinegar can clean brick or stone, is an ingredient in some natural carpet-cleaning recipes, and can be used to clean out the metallic taste in coffeepots and to shine windows without streaking. Vinegar is diluted with water, but it doesn't have to be. An all-purpose cleaner can be made from vinegar and salt.

If you do use chemical cleaners, I encourage you to wear rubber gloves. This will keep chemicals away from your skin so they are not absorbed into your body. Use cleaning agents in well-ventilated areas so that the fumes do not affect your lungs.

Personal Care Products

Every day, you apply personal products—spraying, brushing, or patting them on your body—all of which may contain chemicals from sources you never considered. We are rubbing chemicals on our faces, applying them to our skin, and spraying them on our hair.

Chemicals such as ammonia, formaldehyde, triclosan, and aluminum chlorohydrate are in antiperspirants and deodorants. The chemical triclosan, which is found in some deodorants, has been found to cause liver damage in laboratory rats.[18]

However, there are some safe alternatives. Some companies have pledged not to use chemicals that are harmful to humans. Visit www.safecosmetics

.org for a list of companies. This site also will help you see which of your products are safe and not safe.

Toluene (a solvent similar to benzene), a common ingredient in perfumes and colognes, may contribute to arrhythmias of the heart as well as nerve damage. One way to avoid this is to apply perfume or cologne to your clothes instead of your skin.

A compound called p-Phenylenediamine (PPD) is used in almost every hair dye on the market—even so-called "natural" and "herbal" products. Usually the darker the color, the higher the concentration of PPD. People can be exposed to PPD through inhalation, skin absorption, ingestion, and skin and/or eye contact. Some studies have suggested a connection between hair dyes and myelodysplasia, multiple myeloma, leukemia and preleukemia, non-Hodgkin's lymphoma, and Hodgkin's disease.[19] To reduce your risk of PPD exposure, I recommend sticking to lighter hair colors. If you must use a darker hair color, I advise using semi-permanent or non-permanent coloring.

Although we may be exposed to unsuspected toxins, another method we can use to detoxify is to exercise regularly. One of the benefits of exercise is that it helps the lymphatic system remove cellular waste. Aerobic exercise can increase lymphatic flow threefold, which means that the body can release three times the amount of toxins with regular aerobic exercise.

Chapter 4

HOW STRESS DEPLETES YOUR BODY

MANY YEARS AGO the pastor of our church sometimes would ask me to address the congregation on health topics. By the time I walked onto the platform I would be drenched in sweat, feeling as if I wanted to run out the nearest exit and disappear into the night so I wouldn't have to face the few hundred people in the audience. Public speaking, the most common phobia, terrified me (ironic, considering how much I've done since then, as well as my appearances on TV and in other venues). I remember my pastor putting his hand on my shoulder one time and saying, "You're perspiring terribly. Is it that hot in here?" I didn't have the guts to tell him I was scared to death to be under the spotlight with him. Those moments of stress and plenty of other hard-earned stress lessons from my own life have taught me a lot about the subject.

Some people go through life stressed. Just driving in heavy traffic stresses them out; so does saying hello to a neighbor or calling to inquire about a bill. That stress reaction, so useful in moments of actual emergency, becomes a self-destruct switch that eventually can lead to exhaustion and disease.

When it comes to stress, it is worth remembering that attitudes cause a stress response. Just as certain negative attitudes trigger a long-term stress response, positive attitudes can relieve stress. They are that powerful. An attitude is a manner of acting, feeling, or thinking that reveals a person's disposition or opinion. I personally like the definition of attitude given by one of America's finest Bible teachers and preachers, John Hagee. He sums up attitude with four statements:

> Your attitude is an inward feeling expressed by outward behavior. Your attitude is seen by all without you saying a word.
>
> Your attitude is the "advance man" of your true self. The roots of your attitude are hidden, but its fruit is always visible.
>
> Your attitude is your best friend or your worst enemy. It draws people to you or repels people from you.
>
> Your attitude determines the quality of your relationships with your husband, your wife, your children, your employer, your friends, and God Almighty.[1]

Thoughts and feelings shape attitude, so it is important first and foremost for a person to identify his or her own thoughts and feelings. Examine whether your outlook helps add to the stress that is an innate part of living in the modern world. What are the attitudes that can trigger a stress response in a person's body? They tend to be criticism, pessimism, impatience, and attitudes that might be described as "pushy," "grumpy," and "contentious." Rudeness and self-centeredness are definitely attitudes that impact the body negatively.

These attitudes, of course, give rise to behaviors that most people hate in others but often do not see in themselves, such as whining, murmuring, grumbling, backbiting, and arguing. Such behaviors are unhealthy. So are complaining, disgruntled, manipulative, or lustful (meaning envious or covetous) attitudes. All are markers of a distorted thought process. People who constantly grumble and complain rarely see the goodness or greatness of God. They are focused on self—on *what* they want, *when* they want it, and *how* they want it. This focus, which can be summed up as an attitude of pride, lies at the root of virtually all sin. It is a preoccupation with *me, myself,* and *I.*

What are some of the attitudes that turn off the stress response? Among them are gratitude, contentment, appreciation, joy, love, and compassion. If you have become preprogrammed to complain or to be critical, pessimistic, grumpy, or impatient, make a decision that you will not continue to hold or display these attitudes. Recognize that the attitudes you have are choices you can make. Stress less and, you will enjoy the benefits.

Stress Can Be Good

Now, not all stress in unhealthy. There is good stress, such as that from a family wedding or a promotion. Stress is also our bodies' natural reaction to a threat or perceived threat. It causes a sudden release of adrenaline and other hormones that cause your blood pressure to go up, your heart to beat faster, and your lungs to take in more air, among other physiologic events. These stress hormones give you extra strength and mental acuity for a few moments, and they empower you to either fight or flee.

However, when the stress response occurs too frequently or goes on long term, those stress hormones that were meant to save your life begin to actually harm you. They can leave you feeling depressed, anxious, and angry, with a low sex drive and predisposed to obesity, type 2 diabetes, high cholesterol, hypertension, and all kinds of illnesses. The same hormones that save your life in an emergency can actually begin to destroy your health if the stress response is not turned off.

The Consequences of Stress

One time the *Wall Street Journal* devoted an entire section of its newspaper to how to live longer. The front-page article of the section said, "Increasingly, researchers are viewing stress—how much stress we face in a lifetime, and how well we cope with it—as one of the most significant factors for predicting how well we age."[2] The article concluded that stress "kills" people as much as or more than poor health habits, such as smoking, drinking alcohol, or not exercising.

Stress is not just a mental problem; it's the cause of many of the diseases and maladies I treat in my medical practice. Many recent studies have demonstrated this. The renowned Nun Study has shown that elevated stress levels inhibit and deteriorate the hippocampus, the part of the brain associated with memory and learning. A smaller hippocampus is a sign of Alzheimer's disease.[3]

Final Exam

Students in one study were shown to be more prone to catch a cold, develop cold sores, or get infections when stressed during final exam week.[4]

A long-term study at the University of London showed that chronic unmanaged mental stress was six times more predictive of cancer and heart disease than cigarette smoking, high cholesterol levels, and elevated blood pressure.[5] In a Mayo Clinic study of people with heart disease, psychological stress was the strongest predictor of future cardiac events.[6]

In one ten-year study people who were not able to manage their stress effectively had a 40 percent higher death rate than those who were "unstressed."[7]

Stress, Strokes, and Sickness

Excessive stress long term can make you obese and unhealthy. In response to long-term stress, the hormone cortisol rises, which can cause the blood pressure to rise, can cause the release of fats and sugar in the bloodstream, and may cause weight gain, elevated triglycerides, high cholesterol, and blood sugar. Cortisol will save your life if you are a prisoner of war (POW) or experiencing famine because it slows your metabolic rate and helps preserve your fat stores. But most of us aren't POWs or experiencing famine, so high cortisol levels usually lead to weight gain.

Stressed-out people also tend to develop brown marks under their eyes and frown lines on their foreheads, around the eyes, and around the mouth. Some even get bulging eyes, a tight jaw, and flared nostrils. Plastic surgeons are cashing in on the stress epidemic, performing facelifts and offering Botox injections and more.

What a Headache!

Americans consume sixteen tons of aspirin every year, much of it due to headaches and pains caused by stress.[8]

Cortisol affects the "control loop" that regulates the sex hormones. Elevated cortisol is associated with a drop in dehydroepiandrosterone (DHEA) and testosterone, which can lead to a decreased sex drive and erectile dysfunction. In women elevated cortisol is associated with lower levels of progesterone and testosterone. During periods of chronic stress progesterone is converted to cortisol in the body, which can lead to a progesterone deficiency. This, in turn, can lead to menstrual problems and premenstrual syndrome (PMS), as well as significant menopausal symptoms, such as hot flashes and night sweats. Levels of estrogen usually become imbalanced in the presence of high cortisol.

Chronic stress also has commonly been associated with depression. Elevated cortisol levels cause an imbalance of neurotransmitters in the brain, notably serotonin and dopamine. Lower levels of serotonin or dopamine are associated with depression as is low norepinephrine levels. In one scientific study, as many as seven out of every ten patients with depression had enlarged adrenal glands, some with glands that were 1.7 times the size of a normal gland in a person who is not depressed.[9] In other words, the adrenal gland had enlarged in response to the demand for more cortisol. The cortisol, in turn, causes an imbalance of these important neurotransmitters.

Excessive stress can predispose a person to develop or aggravate every conceivable affliction. Clearly disease and illness are often the shrapnel wounds from stress. If you want to manage your stress, you must first learn to identify causes of stress.

CAUSES OF STRESS

The causes of stress are all too familiar to most Americans. Trouble with finances, relationships, job problems, health, or sudden traumatic events head the list, followed by a myriad of minor stressors, such as smartphone or tablet troubles, traffic, poor customer service, dirty laundry piling up, cleaning house, driving children to extracurricular activities, ongoing conflict with friends or family members, loneliness, or even aggravating lights or noise near your home.

Stress comes in two categories:

1. Things we can and should control
2. Things we cannot control

I hope the following material will help you learn to cope with stress by winning on those two battlefields. Let me illustrate with two examples.

For a long time I was the king of stress clutter in my home office. I received so much "important" material—books, articles, magazines, journals, videos, and more—that I felt I had to read it all. I couldn't bring myself to throw any of it away. I had stacks everywhere of "indispensable" stuff. A normal desk wouldn't accommodate it, so I had to get a huge table to use for a desk. Then my clutter migrated like "the blob" to the kitchen table. I piled books and articles around the house, even in my bedroom, creating knee-high stacks wherever I went. My wife, Mary, or I would walk into the kitchen, my office, or our bedroom and immediately feel stressed out. Neither of us could stand to be in those places.

Ironically the clutter problem was within my realm of control. One day I took responsibility for my messy domain and tossed out as much stuff as I could bear. What I kept, I filed. I have stuck to that system to this day, and my office, our kitchen, and even our bedroom are organized and pleasant. I took action and reduced my stress.

The Top Ten Stressors

According to a 2010 study by the American Psychological Association, the top ten stressors in America are money, work, the economy, family responsibilities, relationships, personal health concerns, housing costs, job stability, health problems affecting one's family, and personal safety, with 76 percent of the respondents reporting money as a cause of stress.[10]

Still, there are also problems that we can't control. In 2004 we went through three major hurricanes within a period of two months. Naturally I felt pretty stressed out. Not only were we left without electricity for days, but also the temperature was near the boiling point.

My office was closed for a few days after each hurricane. My roof leaked, and rain poured into our living room. It flooded our condo and destroyed most of the carpet. The stench of the garbage piling up was terrible because the garbage trucks couldn't get through due to fallen trees and tree limbs blocking the roads. I would lie in bed thinking, "What if we don't have electricity for weeks, and I'm not able to open my office or pay my bills and then end up in extreme debt? What if it costs a lot to repair the roof and fix the condo? What if I can't find a roofing contractor since so many roofs are damaged?"

After each hurricane these thoughts were running through my mind. That created more stress for myself than the hurricanes caused.

Although each hurricane lasted no longer than a day and left a lot of debris that took a few days to clean up, I continued to stress for weeks afterward. My perceptions were at the root of my stress, and they determined how I saw the situation—positive or negative. Instead of having a grateful attitude, I had a "worrywart" attitude. This emotional habit triggered a continuing release of stress hormones. Even though the traumatic hurricanes had passed, I repeatedly relived the stress in my mind over and over, spewing out stress hormones in the process.

Everybody has to deal with unwanted, uncontrollable stress in their lives—natural disasters, unexpected job loss, the death of a loved one, an accident, or an illness. All of these lie mostly outside our realm of control. They require us to change our perceptions and change our reactions.

When I began to practice mindfulness by enjoying the present moment and to reframe the situations by practicing gratitude, my perceptions and reactions changed. I was able to accept my circumstances. The topic of coping with stress is so important that I wrote an entire book on it, called *Stress Less*.[11] I encourage you to purchase it if stress is a problem for you or someone you love.

Wiping Out Worry

In the last section I mentioned how much worrying I did after the hurricanes that struck Florida in 2004. So if you worry, I understand. Yet worry is pointless. I once heard someone say, "I don't worry anymore. I've been a pallbearer for too many of my friends who did." Every day I encounter patients in my office who tell me they are worried about a wide variety of topics. They say such things as:

- "I'm afraid I'm going to lose my job."
- "I'm worried that I might have cancer."
- "I'm worried that I might develop heart disease or Alzheimer's disease."
- "I'm worried that I might lose my hair."
- "I'm worried that my wife might have an affair."

All I can say is my experience shows the fruitlessness of such behavior—not just because we are usually fretting about nothing, but because worry and anxiety are unhealthy. Both are internal, unpleasant clusters of "nervous" or agitated thoughts and feelings that something unpleasant *may* happen (or already did). Worry and anxiety tend to be related to things we think about, imagine, or perceive. Whether short term or long term, they can become almost a state of mind. Some people worry about everything! In doing so, they raise their stress level.

The terms *anxiety attack* and *panic attack* have now been given to an intense bout of worry or anxiety in which the heart rate increases and a person may hyperventilate, sweat, tremble, feel weak, or have stomach or intestinal discomfort.

Such anxiety can originate with distortional thought patterns. Chronic worriers nearly always have distortional thoughts. The two main distortional thought patterns linked to worry are the "what if...?" thought pattern, which sidetracked me in 2004, and what I call "catastrophizing."

"What if . . . ?"

The most common distortional thought pattern linked to worry is a repetition of "What if...?" questions. People ask questions such as, "What if I get fired?" or "What if I don't finish my project before the deadline?" or "What if I have a heart attack?" or "What if my son becomes an alcoholic?" or "What if the food burns and catches the house on fire?" They never end! The "what if-ers" usually analyze a potentially dangerous situation without ever drawing any conclusions or mapping out any solutions, while nearly always carrying the scenario to its worst possible conclusion.

One of the chronic worriers I treated in years past was Maureen, a hypochondriac. For a while I saw her monthly. While she had hypertension (high blood pressure), she really came to see me so often to ask "what if...?" questions, in hopes of alleviating some of her worry. She knew enough about anatomy and medical conditions to be suspicious of a wide variety of symptoms.

She would ask questions such as:

- "What if that sharp pain in my arm is a symptom of a heart attack?"
- "What if that pain in my abdomen is caused by an abdominal aneurysm?"
- "What if that flutter in my chest is a dangerous arrhythmia?"

Maureen had been to see three different cardiologists who had put her through three different nuclear stress tests, three echocardiograms, two heart catheterizations, and numerous other cardiac tests—at the age of thirty-five! As you may have guessed, there was little likelihood of her having a heart attack or angina. The main reason she had all these tests was because she pressed for them, convinced that she "needed to be sure." The physicians she saw feared that if there was something truly wrong and they didn't order the tests, they might get sued.

When her cardiologists and I finally convinced her that she had a healthy heart and cardiovascular system, she switched diseases. Her questions became, "What if that occasional abdominal discomfort is a cancerous tumor?" or "What if that occasional headache is a sign of a brain tumor?"

Prodded by these new, imaginary worries, Maureen made the rounds of new specialists, who would order various CT scans and MRIs to rule out cancer in various parts of her body. Finally I convinced her that the specialist she really needed to see was a psychiatrist. Maureen agreed to go primarily because her "what if...?" preoccupation had already cost her a marriage, custody of her children, and her job as well as caused bankruptcy!

The psychiatrist placed her on medication and referred her to a cognitive behavioral therapist. Over time the therapist helped Maureen reprogram her thinking, but perhaps the simplest and yet most beneficial thing the therapist did was insist that Maureen wear a thick rubber band around her wrist. She was instructed that each time she found herself thinking or saying, "What if...?" she was to pull the rubber band and let it snap back to her wrist, which brought a little sensation of pain. Over time she reprogrammed herself to get rid of "what if...?" thinking. She went on to remarry and be a wonderful wife and mother.

The "Catastrophizer"

Imaginary worries don't limit themselves. In many ways Abraham—whom the Bible calls the "father" of all who have faith—represents the second kind of "worrywart": the catastrophizer. When famine swept the land where Abraham lived, he went to Egypt with his wife, Sarai, a beautiful woman. Abraham told Sarai that when the Egyptians saw her they would think she was his wife and would kill him so they might have her. Abraham immediately projected the worst possible outcome!

As a result, he asked Sarai to say that she was his sister instead. When Abraham and Sarai arrived in Egypt, this is exactly what happened. Sarai wound up in Pharaoh's harem, and in turn Pharaoh gave Abraham a great quantity of livestock, sheep, oxen, male and female donkeys, male and female servants, and camels. However, the Lord sent great plagues on Pharaoh and his house because of Sarai. Eventually Pharaoh discovered the truth and called Abraham in to ask why he had lied about Sarai. He returned Sarai to Abraham and sent him out of Egypt. (See Genesis 12:10–20.)

This happened a second time when Abraham found himself in the land ruled by Abimelech the king of Gerar. Abraham again introduced his wife as his sister. (By this time God had changed her name from Sarai to Sarah.) The king took Sarah to be one of his wives, but before he could have sexual relations with her, God warned him in a dream that she was Abraham's wife and that he needed to restore her to Abraham. Abimelech did so immediately!

Again, Abraham had "catastrophized" an outcome that wasn't anything close to what God had designed for his life.

Don't be too hard on Abraham, though. He symbolizes what so many of us do. Too many people, it seems, focus on what Jesus told His disciples: "In the world you will have tribulation" (John 16:33). Knowing that tribulation can mean anguish, burdens, troubles, and persecution, they raise every minor hassle and inconvenience to that level. They forget that Jesus immediately followed His "tribulation" statement with these words: "But be of good cheer, I have overcome the world" (John 16:33).

Care Versus Overcare

However, you may say, "I'm not worrying; I'm just concerned. Isn't it right to 'care'?" Yes, it's right to care, but not to overcare. Doc Childre, founder of the HeartMath Institute, coined this term, *overcare*, to describe an emotional state. He says overcare is "simply too much care and concern that leads to worry."[12]

Overcare is one of the main reasons clergy members experience such a high burnout rate.

H. B. London, the longtime "Pastor to Pastors" (he now holds the "Emeritus" designation) for Focus on the Family, has called the pastor an "endangered species." Former denominational executive Dr. David Rambo once "reported that 90 percent of pastors say they are inadequately trained to cope with ministry demands, 80 percent say their ministries have had a negative effect on their families, and 70 percent have a lower self-image than when they started in the ministry."[13] I have heard that more pastors are leaving ministry than entering it.

Personally I believe one reason pastors experience a high burnout rate is because many do not fully count the cost of ministry prior to entering this profession. Many seem to have an idealistic belief that all they need to do is prepare a sermon for Sunday morning. They don't realize that they will be called upon to be a church administrator during the week, even as they visit the sick and conduct funerals and weddings. Many are on call 24/7. Excessive care can easily turn into overcare—taking on too much responsibility for too many people.

The person who is called upon to do too much for too many is a person who soon finds that he or she cannot succeed in helping everybody all the time, and perhaps not even succeed in helping some people some of the time. There's a growing sense of inability, inadequacy, insufficiency...in a word, failure. When overcare exhausts a person's emotional reserves, there doesn't seem to be enough "energy" left to deal with the rest of life's practical issues. People with joy and a relaxed attitude can become irritating—rather than be a joy, they become an added burden. The result is that life seems futile, with no hope for any real change. Overcare can lead to "cease to care."

Indeed, it can even be fatal. I'm reminded of the young girl I knew who received a beautiful flowering plant for her twelfth birthday. She was so excited! She had never taken care of a plant all her own, but she was determined to keep it alive and beautiful. She knew that where she lived in Florida, people often watered their lawns daily, so she began to water her plant daily.

After two weeks, she noticed a couple of leaves turning yellow. She decided she wasn't watering the plant often enough, so she began to water twice a day and to add fertilizer to the water. Within a week, all the leaves had turned yellow. The next week, all the leaves fell off. She killed her plant with overcare.

Some of us do the same thing with our health. We are applying so much worry to our lives in the name of care and concern that we are setting ourselves up for disastrous results that could become deadly results. Don't create more stress for yourself by trying to take on far more than God intended for you to have. Relax! The life you save may be your own.

Matthew 11:28–30 says, "Come to Me, all you who labor and are heavy laden." In other words, all you stressed-out people, Christ will "give you rest," not stress. He said, "Take My yoke upon you and learn from Me, for I am gentle and lowly in heart, and you will find rest for your souls. For My yoke is easy and My burden is light." When Jesus said, "Take My yoke upon you," He was saying, "Take...no thought for the morrow" (Matt. 6:34, KJV).

Stress can wreak havoc on your physical body and emotions. Gaining control over stress and its unpleasant side effects will involve bringing your physical body back to a healthier state. This can be accomplished through trusting in God, and it can be helped with supplements and proper nutrition.

Chapter 5

YOUR WEIGHT AND METABOLISM

I LOVE WATCHING TIME-LAPSE videos. Whether it's a nightly weather report showing the day's cloudscape or a montage of a busy street corner's ebb and flow of people, there is something fascinating about getting to see months, weeks, days, or hours of time condensed into mere seconds.

My interest in this began years ago when I saw a documentary using time-lapse filming to capture the effects of the ocean on the coastline. I sat mesmerized as I watched waves pound away at the rocks, day after day, tide in and tide out. After first glance it appeared the water was not doing anything special. Even after several months and years, the coast essentially looked the same. Yet the documenters proved that had their video been able to track thousands of years—or even billions of years, as some geologists claim—I would have been able to see an entirely different landscape formed. By repeatedly and ceaselessly beating down the shoreline, the ocean was actually wearing down the rocks. Eventually even these seemingly immovable structures could be molded into completely different forms through the power of erosion.

Repeat dieting—often referred to as yo-yo dieting—has a similar effect on our bodies. More specifically it wears down our metabolism. Generally when you yo-yo diet, your muscle mass decreases and your body fat increases. Even without dieting, the average person loses between five and seven pounds of muscle mass every ten years after age thirty-five.[1] When you are a repeat dieter, however, you usually lose even more of this muscle mass. Even on many diets that result in weight loss, approximately half the pounds you lose are fat, and the remainder is usually metabolically active muscle and water. It's hard to stress enough how detrimental this is to gaining sustained control of your weight. Muscle is extremely valuable! In fact, muscle cells burn about seventy times more calories than fat cells, which is why they are so crucial for maintaining weight loss.

Unfortunately each time you hop on and off another diet, you typically lose valuable muscle and regain extra fat. Worse still, you are gradually becoming fatter by dramatically lowering your metabolic rate. Studies show that with every decade of muscle loss, your metabolism also decreases by about 5 percent.[2] In essence, every time you drop out of another diet attempt, you make the next one even more difficult.

To find out how you can stop this cycle and restore your metabolic system, let's first take a look at how metabolism works.

BURN WHILE YOU REST

Metabolism is defined as the chemical processes continuously going on in living cells or organisms that are essential for the maintenance of life.[3] It is actually the sum total of all chemical reactions in the body. Keep in mind that your tissues and organs never take a break. Your heart always pumps, your lungs always take in a breath, your liver never stops with its five hundred different functions—including filtering the blood; removing toxins; processing fats, proteins, and carbohydrates; producing bile; and detoxifying chemicals, toxins, and metabolic waste. Your brain and nervous system, digestive system, immune system, hormones, bones, joints, muscles, every tissue of your body—these all require energy and never stop performing their functions, which all contribute to the metabolic rate.

Since it takes energy for your heart to beat, your lungs to breathe, and all your organs to function properly, the metabolic rate is simply the rate at which you burn calories in a non-active state. When considered over a twenty-four-hour period, this is called the basal metabolic rate (BMR) or resting metabolic rate. You typically burn about 75 percent of your calories during a state of rest.

There are several factors that influence your metabolic rate, including your stress level, muscle mass, eating behaviors, appetite hormones, food choices, and activity level. One of the biggest is skipping meals. When you do not eat for more than twelve hours, your metabolic rate goes down by about 40 percent. This sets you up for weight gain, which is compounded when you consume high-sugar, high-carbohydrate, high-fat foods since your body will not burn as many calories in this lowered metabolic state. This is also why eating a healthy breakfast (literally breaking a "fast" through the night as you sleep) is so essential. Individuals who eat breakfast are typically leaner than those who skip breakfast because their metabolic rate is generally higher.

As you might guess, body fat is not metabolically active tissue. Muscle tissue, on the other hand, is extremely metabolically active. The more muscle you have, the higher your metabolic rate will be. The more fat you have, the slower your metabolic rate will be. Think of this another way: it takes far more energy to maintain a pound of muscle than a pound of fat. A good way to increase your metabolic rate is by increasing your muscle mass and decreasing your body fat.

EASIER SAID THAN DONE

For those who have struggled with too much weight for years, many have heard this oversimplified solution: "Losing weight isn't rocket science. All it takes is eating less and exercising more." I've had plenty of obese patients who wanted to wring the necks of all the well-meaning but insensitive people who offer this as a word of "advice." As if these patients had never tried!

The truth is, that formula for weight loss is spot-on. To shed pounds, we do need to eat less and exercise more. But what happens when doing these things doesn't work? What do you do when you have followed every diet and exercise program to the tee and still haven't seen any results?

If this describes you, first let me remind you that you are not alone. As we explore the various reasons why people get stuck in their efforts to lose weight, you will see that many of these factors are reaching epidemic proportions. If you suffer from one or more of these factors, you're accompanied by millions of others—and the club is growing. Second, know that you may be metabolically compromised. All that means is that your metabolism is sluggish and has yet to recover. Somehow—usually through chronic dieting and binge eating—it has been worn down to the point of barely working, which means your body isn't burning fuel the way it should be.

Breathing Test: The Best Way to Measure Your BMR

A routine pulmonary lab test, called indirect calorimetry, can measure oxygen consumption, carbon dioxide production, and respiratory exchange rate. This provides accurate and useful information in providing a detailed picture of the body's metabolic processes at rest.[4]

This can happen for a myriad of reasons. But the overall result is that your body gets locked into *storing* fat rather than *burning* it. Sadly, many obese and metabolically compromised Americans are unaware of the everyday factors that have contributed to their condition. With that in mind, let's examine some of the major factors that can severely affect your metabolic rate.

Avoid Starvation Mode

When you excessively restrict calories and your caloric intake drops below your BMR, you have just entered the starvation zone. Simply put, all your organs and tissues must get their daily calories. When they do not, your brain thinks you are starving and begins to lower your metabolism to conserve energy so you can survive. This is a normal physiologic response.

Unfortunately many diets fail to recognize this and instead go against nature—and we all know who wins that matchup. When you intentionally starve yourself, you not only disrupt your body's natural eating cycle, but you also significantly lower your metabolic rate and disrupt your appetite hormones. I have had many patients complain to me how they have spent entire days eating nothing but two ounces of chicken and a dry salad, yet they still cannot lose weight. Then, after eating just a single baked potato, they suddenly gain a pound. Sound familiar?

Don't Skip Out!

When you don't eat sugar or starches for more than twenty hours, the glycogen (stored sugar) supply in your liver and muscles eventually becomes depleted, causing the liver to break down proteins from muscles and other tissues in a replenishment effort. Because the liver is unable to provide adequate amounts of sugar using this method, you end up feeling fatigued, lethargic, forgetful, spacey, shaky, and lightheaded. This also can trigger the tremendous sugar and starch cravings many people experience in the mid- to late afternoon.

This can be frustrating if you have strictly adhered to the latest fad diet, but what must be understood is the real harm of skipping meals. When you do not eat, your brain interprets your actions as a famine. The appetite hormone ghrelin rises and unleashes a ravenous appetite. It simply does the natural thing and locks into self-protection mode by signaling your metabolism to slow down in order to conserve energy. Without knowing it, you have then turned on the starvation response. You can imagine, then, what effect repeatedly doing this has on your body. Many dieters have reset their metabolic rate time and time again, and the result has been like a stove that no longer functions on high settings but instead only simmers. Though these dieters' internal fires burn, they cannot burn hot enough for them to lose weight.

Chronic Stress

In chapter 4 I discussed the ways stress depletes your body, but I didn't include the observation that chronic stress also lowers the metabolic rate. Our bodies are designed to secrete two stress hormones when we are stressed: epinephrine and cortisol. A "fight-or-flight" hormone, epinephrine works immediately by racing through our bodies when triggered by such stressors as an emergency, running late for an appointment, or an argument with a spouse. When our bodies are unable to fight or flee, we become like rush-hour commuters stuck in bumper-to-bumper traffic on the interstate—we are left literally stewing in our own stress juices.

Epinephrine revs up the stress response by raising our blood pressure and increasing both our heart rate and our breathing. When the perceived stress is over, the epinephrine level typically drops back to normal.

Cortisol, on the other hand, works more slowly, giving us stamina to cope with long-term stress. However, when the stress response becomes stuck as a result of long-term stress, the ongoing elevation of cortisol causes the body to continually release sugar into the bloodstream from glycogen. Glycogen is simply stored sugar, generally held in the liver and muscles. When glycogen is released into the bloodstream, it causes insulin levels to rise, which in turn lowers the blood sugar. Low blood sugar causes more cortisol to be released, leading to weight gain. Excessive insulin also causes the body to store fat in adipose tissue, while also preventing the body from releasing fat from the tissues, even during exercise. In other words, stress programs us for fat storage and contributes significantly to insulin resistance.

Elevated cortisol levels also can cause the body to burn muscle tissue as fuel. Cortisol is a catabolic hormone, which means it causes the body to break down muscle to produce energy, leading to an even lower metabolic rate. As any weightlifter knows, muscle tissue is pricey fuel; we sacrifice our metabolic rate when we burn muscle tissue as fuel. Cortisol is the only hormone that increases as we age.

Certain foods and beverages will raise cortisol levels, including everyday items, such as caffeinated beverages and coffee. In fact, drinking two cups of coffee raises your cortisol levels by approximately 30 percent within a single hour. I am not recommending that you stop drinking coffee—it does have health benefits—but I do recommend you not drink more than two cups a day.

Eating excessive amounts of sugar, white bread, and other high-glycemic foods without the proper ratio of protein, fats, and fiber can cause hypoglycemic episodes, which are bouts with low blood sugar that also raise cortisol levels. Whenever your blood sugar drops, your body is naturally signaled to increase cortisol production. Another way this can happen is through food allergies and sensitivities and by skipping meals and snack times.

The Challenge of Age

Getting older ushers in many health changes, including losing muscle and gaining fat. As we age, not only do we lose muscle mass, but also most people experience decreased levels of hormones—particularly anabolic hormones, which help build muscle and include testosterone, dehydroepiandrosterone (DHEA), and growth hormone. This hormone imbalance can severely stunt any weight-loss efforts.

Among women, this is often seen when they produce either too much or too little estrogen. Both can cause weight gain, particularly in the abdomen, hips, and thighs. Estrogen in the form of birth control pills or hormone replacement therapy commonly causes weight gain. At the same time, many postmenopausal women often chalk up their "menopots" to a lack of estrogen, when in fact it may be due to too much estrogen. In general the more body fat you have, the more estrogen you make. And the more estrogen you make, the more body fat you have; it's a vicious cycle.

Belly Fat and Estrogen

Did you know that belly fat actually produces estrogen? It's true. High levels of estrogen may lead to gynecomastia (enlarged breast tissue in men) and continual weight gain, especially in the hips, waist, and thighs.

This is also the reason why so many obese men have enlarged breasts—their fat cells are simply making too much estrogen. Yes, men have estrogen, just as women have testosterone. In fact, both men and women can struggle with weight gain as a result of low testosterone. Understand that hormones need to be balanced to improve the metabolic rate, build muscle, and burn fat—all of which, of course, affect your weight.

GENDER DIFFERENCES

Women typically have a higher percentage of body fat and lower metabolic rate than men. Although there is currently no consensus on a specific "healthy" range of body fat percentage, and ranges vary according to age, most studies indicate a good goal for women is to keep their body fat under 30 percent. For women, obese is defined as a body fat percentage—not body mass index (BMI)—greater than 33 percent; 31–33 percent is borderline. For men, that goal is less than 20 percent. For men, obese is defined as greater than 25 percent; 21–25 percent is borderline.[5]

By design, women have a lower metabolic rate than men because they typically carry an extra 7 percent to 8 percent of fat on them, even at a healthy weight. Add to this that a woman's metabolic rate declines at the rate of approximately 5 percent per decade of life, beginning at age twenty.

Sit or Get Fit?

Obese people sit down an average of 152 minutes more each day than more slender individuals.[6]

Hazards of Inactivity

Sedentary individuals have a significant loss of muscle mass with aging. I stated earlier that adults naturally lose five to seven pounds of muscle every ten years after age thirty-five just by aging, and as you might guess, inactivity further accelerates this process. The less active we are, the more body fat we keep—and naturally the more muscle we lose. By age sixty most people have lost about twenty-eight pounds of muscle and replaced most of that with much more fat.

I have found this to be especially true among women. I check body fat measurements on all my weight-loss patients and have commonly encountered women with 50 percent body fat or more. It is extremely rare to find this among male patients. Most of these cases have been a result of combining gender with a lack of exercise and metabolic compromise. Obviously women have the disadvantage of carrying a higher percentage of body fat and generally will not lose weight as fast as men. Because of this it is even more important that they be educated about the effects exercise has on metabolism, as well as understanding the unique challenges they face. Remaining sedentary simply compounds the situation and increases their chances of obesity.

Genetic Factors

Though it can easily become an excuse for being overweight, your genetic blueprint greatly influences your metabolic rate. Numerous studies have shown that adopted children rarely resemble the weights of their adoptive parents. Instead, they mimic their biological parents' weight. Too often, however, these individuals use this "genetic card" to account for their obesity and become resigned to this condition for the remainder of their lives. I have found that not to be the case and have seen many of these individuals boost their metabolic rate and lose weight by following a commonsense program of exercise and healthy eating.

Medication Gain

Certain medications can lower your metabolic rate and cause weight gain. These include birth control pills, hormone replacement therapy, prednisone and other steroids, various antidepressants, antipsychotic medications, lithium, insulin and insulin-stimulating medications, cholesterol-lowering medications, some anticonvulsant medications, some antihistamines, and certain blood pressure pills, such as beta-blockers. Ironically many physicians treat diseases caused by obesity, such as hypertension, diabetes, depression, and elevated cholesterol, with the very medications that lower the metabolic rate and result in more weight gain. That is why I typically use vitamins, supplements, and other nutrients as part of the solution for treating obesity-associated problems.

THYROID PROBLEMS

A low or sluggish thyroid also can cause a decreased metabolic rate, though this is often an overlooked problem to the weight-loss equation. I have seen hundreds of cases in which patients reached the end of their rope after adhering to every diet under the sun but never losing weight, only to discover their thyroid was prohibiting them from making progress. Thyroid blood tests should be checked on a regular basis to ensure that the thyroid is functioning normally.

Although men can develop thyroid disease as well, the overwhelming majority of those suffering from thyroid issues are women. An estimated thirteen million American women have some kind of thyroid dysfunction.[7] The sad part is that many of them do not even know it and struggle with weight loss (along with other issues) their entire lives. Researchers say that about 10 percent of younger women and 20 percent of women over age fifty regularly experience mild thyroid problems that impact their weight, attitude, and overall health.[8]

As you can see, there are numerous factors that affect metabolism. One key to keeping yours at a healthy level is avoiding fad diets as you develop a reasonable exercise and activity plan.

Obesity is not helped by the lack of nutrients in our foods. Natural substances and supplements can promote health and vitality as you defeat obesity in your life. Now, continue with me to part 2, where I review the building blocks of good health.

PART II

THE BUILDING BLOCKS OF HEALTH

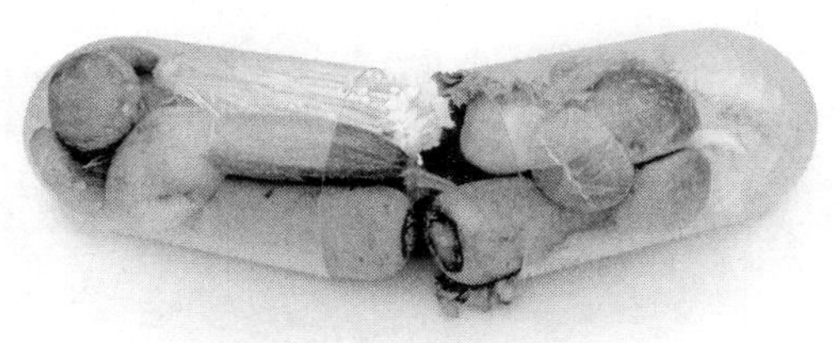

Chapter 6

AN ALPHABET OF NUTRITION: VITAMINS A, C, D, E, K

MOST PEOPLE HAVE the misconception that vitamins will give them instant energy. Vitamins are not pep pills. *Vitamin* literally means "vital amine," and they are indeed needed for many biological processes, including growth, digestion, mental alertness, and resistance to infection. Vitamins enable your body to use carbohydrates, fats, and proteins, and they speed up chemical reactions. Vitamins and minerals are *not optional* for your health. They are at the *very foundation* of your health.

Lack of Nutrients

Most Americans don't get even basic amounts of recommended vitamins and minerals. Here are the fast facts on the vitamins and minerals most Americans lack, what those nutrients do, where they are found, and what happens when you don't get enough of them.

Vitamin A

An estimated 44 percent of Americans are lacking adequate intake of vitamin A,[1] which protects us against cancer and heart disease, prevents night blindness and other eye problems, helps the skin repair itself, and helps in the formation of bones and teeth. Vitamin A is important for the immune system, protecting us against colds, the flu, and infections of the kidneys, bladder, lungs, and mucous membranes.

Beta-carotene is converted in the body to vitamin A and is found in carrots, apricots, leafy greens, garlic, kale, papayas, peaches, red peppers, and sweet potatoes.[2] The recommended daily intake for most adults is 2,300–3,000 international units (IU) daily (an IU is a unit of measurement used in pharmacology and is based on the biological activity of the substance being measured). Lactating women need 4,000 IU a day. Children need only 1,000–2,000 IU daily.[3] Be careful not to go overboard when taking vitamin A. Excessive amounts of vitamin A may lead to liver damage.[4] Dosages greater than 10,000 IU a day of vitamin A were reported in the *New England Journal of Medicine* to have probably been responsible for one out of fifty-seven birth defects in the United States. However, this does not refer to beta-carotene or other carotenoids.[5] Women who are at risk for becoming pregnant should keep their supplemental vitamin A levels below 5,000 IU or choose carotenoids instead of vitamin A.[6] Also, carotenoids, such as beta-carotene, are safer than vitamin A because the body will convert beta-carotene to vitamin A without producing vitamin A in toxic amounts.[7]

The chart below gives some food sources for vitamin A and beta-carotene:[8]

SOURCES OF VITAMIN A		SOURCES OF BETA-CAROTENE	
FOOD	AMOUNT OF VITAMIN A	FOOD	AMOUNT OF BETA-CAROTENE
Spinach, ¼ cup, boiled	5,729 IU	Carrots, boiled, ½ cup slices	13,418 IU
Milk, fortified skim, 1 cup	500 IU	Carrot, raw, 7 inches	8,666 IU
Cheese, cheddar, 1 oz.	249 IU	Cantaloupe, cubed, 1 cup	5,411 IU
Black-eyed peas, boiled, 1 cup	1,305 IU	Spinach, raw, 1 cup	2,813 IU
Broccoli, boiled, ½ cup	1,208 IU	Mango, sliced, 1 cup	1,262 IU
		Peach, 1 medium	319 IU

Lack of vitamin A in your body can cause or be associated with dry hair and skin, dry eyes, poor growth, frequent colds, skin disorders, sinusitis, insomnia, fatigue, and respiratory infections.[9]

Vitamin C

An estimated 50 percent of Americans are lacking adequate intake of vitamin C.[10] Vitamin C helps form collagen, a protein that gives structure to—and maintains—bones, cartilage, muscle, and blood vessels. It also helps heal wounds. The adequate intake is 90 mg per day for adult men and 75 mg for adult women.[11] Common sources include:[12]

FOOD	AMOUNT OF VITAMIN C
Broccoli, cooked, ½ cup	50 mg
Cantaloupe, ½ cup	35 mg
Guava, 1 medium	165 mg
Orange, 1 medium	60 mg
Papaya, 1 medium	95 mg
Red bell pepper, ½ cup	95 mg
Strawberries, ½ cup	45 mg

I recommend a four-ounce glass of fresh-squeezed orange juice every day with the pulp added to it. Vitamin C deficiency causes weakness, fatigue, swollen gums, nosebleeds, and in extreme cases, scurvy.[13] During stress there are higher requirements for vitamin C. It is also reported to reduce the risk of cataracts and retinal damage, increase immune function, and decrease heavy metal toxicity. Increased intake of vitamin C is linked to a reduced risk of cancer of the cervix, stomach, colon, and lungs. It also reduces low-density lipoprotein (LDL) oxidation, which causes plaque buildup in arteries, and it supports healthy blood pressure.[14]

Some people are allergic to vitamin C since the majority of vitamin C comes from corn. You also can find vitamin C-buffered corn-free capsules in health food stores. Instead of deriving vitamin C from corn, these corn-free products derive vitamin C from such sources as the sago palm.

Vitamin D

Approximately 50 percent of the general population is deficient in vitamin D, though that number increases for people of color and the elderly.[15] Vitamin D is required for your body to absorb calcium and phosphorus. It is critically important for growth and for the normal development of bones and teeth.[16] It may protect against prostate and breast cancer. The higher the vitamin D levels in the blood, the lower the risk for colon and colorectal cancers.[17]

But vitamin D deficiency is common among young women (only 20 to 40 percent get the amounts they need) and in people over fifty, particularly women, for whom vitamin D deficiency is epidemic.[18] Very few people overall get enough vitamin D (400 IU) from their diet alone.[19] Sun exposure is the most important source of vitamin D because the skin synthesizes vitamin D in response to UV rays. Most people need only ten to fifteen minutes of direct sun exposure twice a week, without sunscreen, to meet their vitamin D requirement.[20] However, few doctors recommend this since it may increase the risk of skin cancer for some individuals.

There are few good food sources of vitamin D. Cod liver oil offers a whopping 1,360 IU per tablespoon. I usually don't recommend cod liver oil because it may contain some toxins. It also usually has to be over-processed, thus rendering it unstable, and it may contain a higher percentage of oxidized fats.

Three ounces of cooked salmon gives 447 IU. And a cup of milk fortified with vitamin D gives up to 124 IU.[21] Vitamin D_3 is the active form of vitamin D. In its active form vitamin D enhances the absorption of calcium from the small intestines. Even though the recommended dose of vitamin D for adults is 400–800 IU a day, the National Osteoporosis Foundation recommends 800–1,000 IU for those over fifty.[22] I check vitamin D levels on all of my patients, and approximately 90 percent of my patients are initially low in vitamin D_3. I place most of my patients on 2,000–5,000 IU of vitamin D_3 a day.

Vitamin D deficiency is associated with osteoporosis and hip fractures. In a review of women with osteoporosis hospitalized for hip fractures, 50 percent were found to have signs of vitamin D deficiency.[23]

Vitamin E

Research shows that 93 percent of Americans have inadequate intakes of vitamin E,[24] which decreases free-radical damage of lipid membranes and protects the heart, blood vessels, and tissues of the breast, liver, eyes, skin, and testes. Vitamin E decreases blood clotting, which further reduces the risk of heart disease. Most people get vitamin E from vegetable oil products such as salad dressings, though cold-pressed vegetable oils (such as extra-virgin olive oil) are generally highest in vitamin E. (Most vegetable oils are heat processed.) You also can get vitamin E from dark green leafy vegetables, legumes, nuts, seeds, whole grains, brown rice, corn meal, eggs, milk, oatmeal, and wheat germ. Common sources include the following:[25]

FOOD	AMOUNT OF VITAMIN E
Wheat germ oil, 1 Tbsp.	20.3 mg (about 30 IU)
Almonds, dried, 1 oz.	6.72 mg (about 10 IU)
Sweet potato, 1 medium	5.93 mg (about 9 IU)

I recommend the natural vitamin E, which contains all eight forms of vitamin E: alpha-, beta-, delta-, and gamma-tocopherol, and alpha-, beta-, delta-, and gamma-tocotrienol. The names of all types of vitamin E begin with either "d" or "dl." The "d" is the natural form, and the "dl" is the synthetic form, which comes from petroleum. The synthetic form has only about 50 percent of the activity of natural vitamin E.[26] But tremendous confusion and even controversy have surrounded vitamin E since its discovery in 1922. One recent study concluded that in patients with vascular disease or diabetes, the long-term supplementation with the natural source vitamin E (400 IU) does not prevent cancer or cardiovascular events and may actually increase the risk for heart failure.[27] That conclusion had unfortunate consequences because most Americans already lack sufficient amounts of this important nutrient. Some doctors warned their patients not to take vitamin E in a supplement.

The study also ignored the benefits of vitamin E. A different study showed that men who take 50 IU a day, as opposed to the recommended daily value of 30 IU, had 41 percent fewer deaths from prostate cancer than those who did not receive supplemental vitamin E.[28] That's a significant benefit.

One form of vitamin E, gamma-tocopherol, is extremely important. One study found that men with the highest concentration of gamma-tocopherol had a fivefold lower risk of developing prostate cancer than men with the lowest levels.[29] Gamma-tocopherol also may protect one from developing colorectal cancer and Alzheimer's disease.

Prolonged vitamin E deficiency eventually may cause severe neurological complications, including unsteady gait, loss of muscle coordination, muscle weakness, peripheral neuropathy, and diminished reflexes. It also can cause infertility, menstrual problems, miscarriages, and shortened red blood cell life span.

Vitamin Shortage

According to the US Department of Agriculture (USDA), just over one in four Americans meet their adequate intake of vitamin K.

Vitamin K

Studies suggest that 73 percent of Americans do not get adequate intake of vitamin K,[30] which is important in blood clotting, for bone mineralization, and in helping to regulate cellular growth.[31] The daily reference intake for vitamin K for men age nineteen and above is 120 mcg. For women in that age bracket it is 90 mcg.[32] Vitamin K is found in:[33]

FOOD	AMOUNT OF VITAMIN K
Turnip greens, cooked, ½ cup	426 mcg
Broccoli, cooked, ½ cup	110 mcg
Kale, raw, 1 cup	113 mcg
Spinach, raw, 1 cup	145 mcg

Most of your body's supply of vitamin K is synthesized by the friendly bacteria in your intestines. But when you take antibiotics, you increase your need for vitamin K. The antibiotics kill many of the good bacteria, and as a result, the remaining good bacteria cannot produce adequate amounts of vitamin K.[34]

Vitamin K deficiency is associated with easy bruising and bleeding and increased risk of osteoporosis. Vitamin K_2 has been shown to be supportive in preventing calcification or hardening in the arteries.[35] The presence of vitamin K in green leafy vegetables may be one reason vegetarians have a lower incidence of kidney stones.[36] Vitamin K_2 has been shown to lower the risk of coronary heart disease; it also may increase bone density for those with osteoporosis. Vitamin K_2 has been shown to keep more of the calcium in bones, where it is needed, and keep it out of the arteries, where it can form calcified plaque.[37] These vitamins, and many others, are essential to good health and long life. Maintaining long-term deficiencies of any of them is like asking your car to do its job without the proper fuel. In the rest of this section I will be looking at the B vitamins, minerals, antioxidants, phytonutrients, and healthy fats. Remember, you need a balanced diet and supplementation to achieve the kind of optimal health that will carry you through life with a smile on your face and a spring in your step.

Chapter 7

THE B VITAMINS: NUTRITION'S FIRST FAMILY

THE B VITAMINS include thiamine, riboflavin, niacin, pantothenic acid, folic acid, vitamin B_6, vitamin B_{12}, and biotin. For years known as the "stress-relief vitamins," they are also important for optimal immune function. The B-vitamin family provides the greatest benefit when supplemented together, such as with a balanced B complex. Some B vitamins even require other B vitamins for activation. A comprehensive multivitamin should have adequate doses of B-complex. I recommend taking either a multivitamin with B complex or a B-complex vitamin one to two times a day.

The recommended daily intake for B vitamins is rather low, in my opinion. Therefore, I recommend for my patients 5–50 mg of vitamin B_1 (thiamine), 5–50 mg of vitamin B_2 (riboflavin), 20–100 mg of vitamin B_3 (niacin), 10–100 mg of vitamin B_5 (pantothenic acid), and 2–50 mg of vitamin B_6 (pyridoxine). I also recommend 400 mcg of folic acid, 20–200 mcg vitamin B_{12} (methylcobalamin), and 300–600 mcg B_7 (biotin).

The B vitamins are especially important for elderly individuals, since B vitamins are not absorbed as well as you age. They are associated primarily with brain and nervous system function and are used in the production of adenosine triphosphate (ATP). Deficiency in any or all of them is commonly associated with fatigue and sleep disturbances, eventually resulting in atrophy of the adrenal glands.

Except for vitamin B_{12}, the other B vitamins are plentiful in a diet that includes a mix of vegetables, dairy products, and whole grains. Foods of animal origin are also good sources of all the Bs (including vitamin B_{12}). Getting enough vitamin B_{12} may be particularly problematic for vegetarians; this B vitamin is particularly essential for pregnant mothers since it affects a baby's developing blood supply and nervous system. Prenatal vitamin formulations also provide a healthy and balanced dose of the B-complex vitamins.

To review the key B vitamins, read below.

THIAMINE (B_1)

Vitamin B_1, also known as thiamine, is vital for energy, metabolism, growth, and the function of cells. It also may improve cardiovascular health. Thiamine occurs naturally in many foods, including whole grains and meats. Heating foods containing thiamine reduces the thiamine content in the food, and more is lost in water used to cook the food in since this vitamin is water soluble. The recommended amount of thiamine is 1.2 mg for men age nineteen and over, and 1.1 mg for women age nineteen and over. Most Americans do not have a vitamin B_1 deficiency, but it is not unheard of. People with diabetes and the elderly, for instance, are more likely to be deficient in thiamine.[1]

Riboflavin (B_2)

Vitamin B_2, also known as riboflavin, is available in foods as well as supplements. Foods containing riboflavin include eggs, organ meats, green vegetables, and milk. Riboflavin helps with growth, development, function of cells, and converting food into energy. It is best to consume riboflavin in smaller amounts because the body does not absorb a large dosage well. It is recommended for men age nineteen and over to consume 1.3 mg of riboflavin a day, while women need 1.1 mg. Pregnant or breastfeeding women need slightly more—1.4 mg and 1.6 mg, respectively. A deficiency in riboflavin is not common. However, athletes who are vegetarians, vegans, and pregnant or nursing women have a higher chance of experiencing a deficiency.[2]

Niacin (B_3)

Vitamin B_3, also called niacin, is necessary for good health. It can help cholesterol levels—both raising good cholesterol and lowering bad cholesterol—as well as limit the risk of cardiovascular disease. It potentially may help with Alzheimer's disease, diabetes, and more, but more research is needed to verify these claims. Taking too much niacin may be dangerous to your health and may inflame the liver, so talk with your doctor before supplementing with it. Vitamin B_3 is found in some foods, including green vegetables, meat, and eggs. Women need 14 mg of niacin daily, while men need 16 mg. This number is slightly higher for pregnant and breastfeeding women. Pregnant women need 18 mg, while nursing women need 17 mg.[3]

Pantothenic Acid (B_5)

Pantethine is the active, stable form of pantothenic acid, otherwise known as vitamin B_5. It is important for maintaining a healthy thymus gland and for antibody production. It can be used to lower low-density lipoprotein (LDL) cholesterol and triglyceride levels while increasing high-density lipoprotein (HDL) levels. It is believed that pantethine inhibits the production of cholesterol and accelerates the breakdown of fatty acids in the body.

Pantothenic acid is known as the "anti-stress vitamin" because it plays such a vital role in the production of adrenal hormones. A deficiency of pantothenic acid, while rare, is serious and leads to a decreased resistance to stress.[4] Pantothenic acid provides critical support for the adrenal glands as it responds to stress; adequate supplementation is crucial for the health of adrenal glands in most people. I believe vitamin B_5 is the most important B vitamin for restoring and maintaining adrenal function. I typically place patients with adrenal fatigue on 250–500 mg two times a day.

Pantothenic acid also can be found in salmon, yeast, vegetables, dairy, eggs, grains, and meat.

Pyridozine (B_6)

Vitamin B_6 is vital for the utilization of amino acids (which are the building blocks for proteins). A vitamin B_6 deficiency often is marked by depression, irritability, nervousness, muscle weakness, dermatitis, slow learning, numbness, and cramping in the extremities. The nervous system requires this vitamin. It also is needed for normal brain functions and to produce dopamine, serotonin, and gamma-aminobutyric acid (GABA). These are very important neurotransmitters for promoting feelings of well-being, relaxation, and calmness.

Vitamin B_6 is especially important for women using oral contraceptives (birth control pills) and experiencing bouts of depression, irritability, moodiness, fatigue, and decreased sex drive. Many of these symptoms can be reversed with this supplement.[5] Food sources include lentils, lima beans, soybeans, sunflower seeds, bananas, avocados, buckwheat, and brewer's yeast.

In addition, vitamin B_6 is crucial for nursing mothers. It plays an integral role in the functioning of the nervous and immune systems. The risk of B_6 deficiency is higher in babies who are exclusively breast-fed beyond six months of age. If your breast-fed baby shows little or no interest in solid foods, you can ensure adequate amounts of B_6 go into your breast milk by eating foods rich in B_6, as well as taking a quality multivitamin or prenatal vitamin.

Although vitamin B_6 performs many functions in your body, studies show that 28 percent of women nineteen years of age and older do not have adequate intake of this vitamin.[6] It is necessary for protein metabolism as well as red blood cell metabolism. The nervous and immune systems need it to function efficiently. It helps increase the amount of oxygen carried to your tissues, and it helps keep your blood sugar level in a normal range. It is very important in the synthesis of the neurotransmitters serotonin and dopamine.[7] Vitamin B_6 is found in fortified cereals, fish, poultry, red meat, and some produce.

Here is a list of foods and the amount of vitamin B_6 they contain[8]:

FOOD	AMOUNT OF VITAMIN B_6
Potato, boiled, 1 cup	0.40 mg
Banana, medium	0.43 mg
Chicken, roasted, 3 ounces	0.50 mg

FOOD	AMOUNT OF VITAMIN B_6
Brussels sprouts, 1 cup	0.28 mg
Collard greens, boiled, drained, 1 cup	0.24 mg
Sunflower seeds, kernels only, dried, ¼ cup	0.47 mg
Bell peppers, raw, 1 cup	0.27 mg
Broccoli pieces, cooked, 1 cup	0.31 mg
Watermelon, 1 cup	0.10 mg
Avocado, raw, 1 cup, sliced	0.39 mg

Signs of vitamin B_6 deficiency include skin irritation, headaches, sore tongue, depression, confusion, convulsions, anemia, and premenstrual syndrome (PMS). If you are deficient in vitamin B_6, B_{12}, or folic acid, then levels of homocysteine, a toxic amino acid, may rise in the blood. Homocysteine has a toxic effect on the cells lining the arteries, causing plaque to form on the artery lining, and high levels may bring issues such as cardiovascular disease, Alzheimer's, and osteoporosis.[9] However, taking excess vitamin B_6 (100 mg or more) can lead to peripheral neuropathy so use caution when choosing a B-complex vitamin, and do not choose B-100 complex.

BIOTIN (B_7)

Vitamin B_7, also known as biotin, is important in many areas of the body. It can help skin, nerves, the digestive tract, and metabolism. There is some evidence that it may help lower the blood sugar and also decrease insulin resistance in those with type 2 diabetes. Biotin can be found naturally in whole wheat, eggs, dairy, salmon, and more. However, it can be gained through supplements as well. Adults age nineteen and up need 30 mcg of biotin each day.[10]

FOLIC ACID (B_9)

Folic acid, also known as vitamin B_9, is important for optimal function of T-cells and B-cells. It is important for brain function as well as mental health. B vitamins, particularly folic acid, help keep homocysteine levels in the normal range.[11] Folic acid may even help keep the heart healthy and reduce the incidence of heart disease. Some researchers have suggested that an increase of folic acid intake could potentially prevent an estimated 13,500 deaths from cardiovascular disease each year.[12] The active form of folic acid is methyltetrahydrofolate (MTHF). In fact, a new medicine for depression is Deplin or MTHF.

Folic acid deficiency is especially common in alcoholics, indigent populations, the elderly, and individuals with malabsorption disorders. One study conducted at the Massachusetts General Hospital in Boston found that people with low folate levels were more likely to have melancholic depression and were significantly less likely to respond to Prozac, a very popular antidepressant medication.[13]

Folic acid may be found in several foods. Leafy green vegetables are particularly high in the vitamin, as are beans, dairy products, poultry, and more. Adults age nineteen and over need 400 mcg of folic acid per day. However, it is important for pregnant women to get more to limit the risk of certain birth defects. It is recommended that pregnant women consume 600 mcg of folic acid each day.

Methylcobalamin (B_{12})

Studies suggest that approximately 25 percent of the population has inadequate intake of vitamin B_{12}.[14] A vitamin B_{12} deficiency has been related to peripheral neuropathy, anemia, paresthesias, demyelination of the dorsal columns and corticospinal tract of the spinal cord, depression, dementia, and heart disease. A deficiency also has been associated with low energy, poor memory, problems in thinking, low stomach acid, and elevated homocysteine levels.[15]

A study conducted at Tufts University found that nearly 40 percent of those studied had a B_{12} blood level in "low normal" range, which is where neurological symptoms begin to occur. Individuals between the ages of twenty-six and forty-nine were discovered to have the same high risk for B_{12} deficiency as those over sixty-five.[16]

Vitamin B_{12} is needed by phagocytes—those cells that fight bacteria that cause strep throat and other infections. It is also important for maintaining the myelin sheaths that cover and protect nerve endings. Subclinical or borderline B_{12} deficiency is rather common, especially among the elderly.[17] We know from nutrition-related research that the processing and refining of foods destroys much of the vitamins B_6, B_{12}, and folic acid in them. With so many Americans hooked on highly processed foods, fast foods, and foods containing large amounts of sugar, it is probable that countless American adults are suffering from borderline or frank deficiency in these B vitamins. This may be one reason for the escalation of cardiovascular and stress-related diseases.

Nursing mothers should especially pay attention to getting adequate amounts of B_{12}. This vitamin creates and maintains DNA and RNA (ribonucleic acid), the genetic templates from which our cells are made. A growing baby's body is making new cells rapidly. If B_{12} is not available in adequate supply, growth and development suffer.

Folic acid/folate plays a major role in producing and maintaining new cells. So in addition to vitamin supplements, new mothers should eat plenty of green vegetables, whole grains, and beans.

Chapter 8

DIGGING FOR GOLD: MINERALS AND YOUR BODY

JUST LIKE VITAMINS, minerals are not optional for your health, but help form its very foundation. The human body needs twenty-two essential minerals on a daily basis. Because our soil has become depleted or is lacking in minerals, the food we grow and eat provides less and less of these essential nutrients. Therefore, the vast majority of Americans need to take minerals in supplement form. Many people are deficient in several of these minerals. And just like most Americans don't get even basic amounts of recommended vitamins, they also fail to get enough minerals. Failing to obtain adequate minerals leaves your body deprived and unable to function properly. To paraphrase the prospectors of old: "There's gold in them thar minerals!"

Here are some of the minerals your body needs.

MAGNESIUM

A building block of health, magnesium is needed for protein, fatty acid, and bone formation. Yet 68 percent of Americans aren't consuming enough.[1] Many Americans are woefully lacking in magnesium. As a matter of fact, it is one of the most common deficiencies in the country, especially for the elderly. Why? We drink too much coffee and alcohol, and we eat too many processed foods, all of which rob our bodies of this important mineral.

Magnesium is used in making new cells, in relaxing muscles, and in the clotting of blood. It helps form adenosine triphosphate (ATP), which gives us energy. It assists with over three hundred different enzyme reactions in the body; helps prevent muscle spasm, heart attacks, and heart disease; aids in lowering blood pressure; and eases asthma. It also helps prevent osteoporosis and helps regulate the colon and bowels. The recommended daily amount for the average person from fifteen to fifty years old is 400 mg. Magnesium is found in nuts, seeds, dark green leafy vegetables, grains, and legumes. It is easy to see why many Americans are deficient in this important mineral because many are eating fast foods and junk foods instead of "living foods." Common sources of magnesium include:[2]

FOOD	AMOUNT OF MAGNESIUM
Halibut, cooked, 3 oz.	24 mg
Almonds, dry roasted, 1 oz.	80 mg
Cashews, dry roasted, 1 oz.	74 mg
Spinach, boiled, ½ cup	78 mg

In order to get your recommended daily intake (RDI), you would have to eat about five ounces of almonds every day. If you don't get enough magnesium, you may experience loss of appetite, nausea, and fatigue. If the deficiency worsens, patients may develop muscle weakness, muscle twitches, irregular heartbeat, leg cramps, insomnia, and eye twitches. Symptoms of deficiency also include constipation, headaches, personality changes, and coronary spasms.

Magnesium and Regularity

Your colon needs magnesium to help it undergo peristalsis, which propels food through and out. Most Americans don't get adequate amounts of fiber, magnesium, and water.

Calcium

Your body also requires calcium in relatively large amounts, and many Americans do not consume enough. About 99 percent of your calcium resides in your bones and teeth. The remaining 1 percent circulates in your blood and carries out the critical function of regulating muscle contraction, heart contraction, and nerve function. Calcium gives you strong bones and prevents osteoporosis. It even lowers blood pressure. Some studies suggest that when you get adequate calcium in dietary and supplemental form, you decrease your risk of colon cancer.[3]

Calcium is found in higher amounts in these foods:[4]

FOOD	AMOUNT OF CALCIUM
Yogurt, plain, low-fat, 8 oz.	415 mg
Calcium-fortified soy milk, 8 oz.	299 mg
Turnip greens, boiled, ½ cup	99 mg
Kale, cooked, ½ cup	94 mg
Milk, nonfat, 8 fl. oz.	299 mg
Cheddar cheese, 1½ oz.	307 mg
Tofu, firm, made with calcium sulfate, ½ cup	253 mg
Cottage cheese, 1% milk fat, 1 cup unpacked	138 mg

Children and teens age nine to eighteen need 1,300 mg a day, persons age nineteen to fifty need 1,000 mg a day, men over age fifty need 1,000 mg a day, and women over age fifty need 1,200 mg.[5] The problem is, if you don't consume enough dietary calcium, your body eventually will cannibalize the calcium from the bones to maintain calcium levels in the blood. This can quietly lead to osteopenia and osteoporosis, which literally means "porous bones"—or bones lacking in minerals and mass. Very few women get all the calcium they need from diet, and in old age their skeletons shrink. The first bones to go are the jawbone and the vertebrae in the back, which is why older people lose their teeth and height. Calcium deficiencies also can result in leg cramps, muscle cramps, and even hemorrhaging, blood loss, and anemia (since calcium is essential to blood clotting).[6]

Studies show that more than 75 percent of Americans do not meet the current recommendations for calcium intake.[7] Low calcium intake has become a major public health problem in the United States. At the same time, you do not want to consume too much calcium. A 2013 study from the National Institutes of Health showed that calcium supplementation may increase the risk of heart attack and other cardiovascular disease in men, while other studies have indicated this may be true for both men and women. Regardless, discuss calcium supplementation and its risks and benefits for you with your health care provider.[8] Until further studies confirm that calcium supplementation is not harmful, I have lowered my recommendation for calcium supplementation in women over fifty to 200–250 mg three times a day and in men 200–250 mg two to three times a day. I also place all patients taking calcium supplementation on vitamin K_2 at least 100 mcg a day. This will help to keep the calcium in the bones and out of the arteries.

POTASSIUM

Potassium is a mineral that helps muscles contract, maintains fluid balance, sends nerve impulses, and releases energy from food. Potassium is needed to regulate blood pressure, neuromuscular function, and levels of acidity. Your body needs sodium and potassium to maintain good health. They both help regulate fluids in and out of your body cells. According to a recent report most adults consume excessive amounts of sodium, but many don't consume enough potassium.[9] This is no surprise; processed and fast foods are high in sodium, and fruits and most vegetables are high in potassium. The average American diet is lacking in fruits and vegetables. The Institute of Medicine of the National Academies of Science has issued recommendations for sodium and potassium intake levels. They say that healthy adults between the ages of nineteen and fifty should consume about 1,500 mg of sodium per day and 4,700 mg of potassium.[10]

Potassium Overload?

Fewer than 5 percent of people eat more than their adequate intake of potassium.[11]

Potassium is one of the main electrolytes in the body, along with sodium and chloride. These three electrolytes play a key chemical role in every function of the body.

Reach your recommended daily intake of potassium by adding these foods to your daily menu: fish, potatoes, avocadoes, dried apricots, bananas, citrus juices, dairy products, and whole grains. All are wonderful sources of potassium. The top foods are:[12]

FOOD	AMOUNT OF POTASSIUM
Sweet potato, medium, baked	542 mg
Tomato paste, ¼ cup	669 mg
Beet greens, cooked, ½ cup	654 mg
Yogurt, plain, nonfat, 8 oz.	579 mg
Halibut, cooked, 3 oz.	449 mg
Soybeans, green, cooked, ½ cup	485 mg
Banana, medium	422 mg
Milk, nonfat, 1 cup	382 mg

To put this chart into practical application, the first line means that the average adult would have to eat the equivalent of three baked sweet potatoes daily to get the RDI. Eating five to seven servings of fruits and vegetables a day will usually provide adequate potassium.

At the beginning of this section I mentioned that most adults consume excessive amounts of sodium but not enough potassium. Here's another hazard from eating too much sodium: it may lower your body's store of potassium. Low potassium intake is associated with high blood pressure; irregular heartbeat; wheezing and asthma; weakness; nausea; loss of appetite; altered mental states, including nervousness and depression; dry skin; insomnia; and fatigue.

Iodine

Iodine is a mineral that is essential for proper thyroid function. Without adequate iodine intake, the thyroid gland is unable to make adequate amounts of thyroid hormones. An iodine deficiency can cause hypothyroidism, developmental brain disorders, and goiter (thyroid enlargement). In children hypothyroidism as a result of iodine deficiency can cause stunted growth, mental retardation, and speech and hearing problems.

Even though iodine is not yet recognized as a major deficiency in America, I have found that many of my patients are iodine deficient. Some researchers believe that iodine deficiency is on the rise in the United States. A past issue of the *Journal of Clinical Endocrinology & Metabolism* reported that the percentage of Americans who don't consume enough iodine had more than quadrupled between the late 1970s and the late 1990s.[13]

The reason Americans are consuming less iodine is because—like so many other nutrients that I have already discussed—our soil is deficient in it, especially in inland and mountainous areas. Also, approximately 50 percent of people use salt without iodine, and Americans are cutting down on salt. Breads and pastas no longer contain iodine. Instead, they contain bromide, which behaves like a goitrogen and inhibits iodine binding. Fluoride and chlorine, found in much of our tap water, also inhibit iodine binding.

In addition to the conditions listed above, low iodine is linked to fibrocystic breast disease and cysts of the ovaries, making women more likely to suffer from physical problems as a result of iodine deficiency.[14] Evidence shows that adequate intake of iodine makes a difference in warding off these conditions. Foods that are high in iodine include kelp, dulse, other sea vegetables, potatoes, strawberries, yogurt, and more.

Other Necessary Minerals

These minerals, and many others, are essential to good health and long life. In addition to the minerals I have reviewed, your body needs a few more essential and trace minerals. The first four minerals below—phosphorus, chloride, sulfur, and silicon—are major minerals that you need daily. You need the remaining minerals in smaller quantities.

Phosphorus

The American diet is high in phosphorus, and we do not need to supplement. Adults nineteen and over need approximately 700 mg a day.[15] Phosphorus helps the body produce energy and bone as well as helps the blood deliver oxygen.[16]

Chloride

Americans rarely are deficient in chloride due to their high intake of salt, which is sodium chloride. However, adults aged nineteen to fifty need 2,300 mg per day of chloride.[17] Chloride is necessary in the digestive system, and it helps balance bodily fluids.[18]

Sulfur

This mineral helps form our tissues and activates enzymes. It is also used for manufacturing many proteins, including those forming hair, skin, and muscles. It is a component of insulin and is needed to regulate blood sugar.

Silicon

Essential for skeletal growth and development, silicon plays a role in maintaining connective tissue and bone.

Iron

This mineral forms the oxygen-carrying portion of the red blood cell. Without adequate iron, you may become anemic and tired. Men and post-menopausal women, except those with iron-deficiency anemia, don't need extra iron. Also, iron can be a two-edged sword because excessive amounts can cause oxidative damage to cells and organs. Women aged nineteen to fifty need 18 mg of iron daily, while men need only 8 mg.[19] Both men and women over fifty need 8 mg of iron daily.[20]

Zinc

A very important mineral, zinc is a component of more than three hundred enzymes. It is needed to repair wounds, to improve immunity, to assist in fertility, to maintain vision, and to synthesize proteins. A deficiency of zinc is associated with skin problems, dermatitis, and healing problems. Deficiencies also affect learning and behavior. A simple screening test to help determine if you possibly are deficient in zinc is the zinc tally test. Place a teaspoon of zinc sulfate on your tongue and hold it in your mouth for five to ten seconds. If you do not taste the zinc, which has a bitter flavor, then you are probably lacking zinc.

Copper

A deficiency in copper is related to a decrease in energy production and decline in immune function and mental concentration. Like iron, copper needs to be limited and balanced with zinc because too much copper can cause oxidative damage to your tissues. Both men and women aged nineteen and over need 900 mcg of copper each day.[21]

Manganese

Deficiencies of manganese are associated with weakness, growth retardation, and bone malformations. Men nineteen and older need 2.3 mg of manganese each day. Women need 1.8 mg.[22]

Chromium

Helping to maintain normal blood sugar levels and regulate insulin, chromium also may help control blood sugar in diabetics and patients with hypoglycemia. Men aged nineteen to fifty need 35 mcg, and women need

25 mcg, each day. Over the age of fifty, women need 20 mcg and men need 30 mcg.[23]

Vanadium

Both chromium and vanadium are important in glucose and insulin metabolism. They have a positive effect on normalizing blood sugar for both hypoglycemia and diabetes.

Selenium

This mineral supports your immune system and helps prevent cardiomyopathy—a heart-weakening disease. Both men and women age nineteen and older need 55 mcg of selenium on a daily basis.[24]

Molybdenum

This mineral helps the body use iron, promotes normal growth and development, and may prevent anemia, tooth decay, and impotency. Adults need 45 mcg per day.[25]

Boron

This mineral is essential for normal calcium and bone metabolism. There is no recommended daily value for boron. A diet considered to be high in boron provides approximately 3.25 mg of boron per 2,000 kcal per day. Diets that provide 0.25 mg of boron per 2,000 kcal per day are considered to be low in boron.[26]

Cobalt

You will have plenty of cobalt in your system as long as you take a multivitamin with B_{12}, which is cobalamin.

As you can see, there are many minerals that can improve your health, or be detrimental if you do not consume enough. Look into these minerals and your diet, and see what you may be lacking.

Chapter 9

YOUR NEED FOR ANTIOXIDANTS

LET'S SAY THAT you are a health enthusiast—someone who eats anywhere from five to thirteen servings of fruits and vegetables a day—and take a multivitamin that contains adequate amounts of vitamin E, vitamin C, selenium, and beta-carotene every day. You may believe that such a regimen gives you the antioxidants needed to prevent disease. However, you are most likely not taking the correct antioxidants. While the body produces three main antioxidants, five major antioxidants need to be supplemented.

However, before discussing antioxidants, it is critically important to understand free radicals—how they start and how we can protect ourselves from them. Let's begin by discussing the chemical process of oxidation. When metals such as iron are oxidized, it produces rust. When oxidation occurs on painted surfaces, the paint begins to flake off. When you cut an apple in half, it starts to turn brown within a few minutes because of oxidation. Oxidation also occurs when food spoils, meat rots, and fats rancidify. Free radicals cause oxidation.

Want to Live to Be One Hundred?

Blood levels of antioxidants generally decrease with age. However, Italian researchers discovered that centenarians (individuals one hundred years of age or older) had significantly higher blood levels of vitamins A and E than younger counterparts. The Italian researchers concluded, "It is evident that healthy centenarians show a particular profile in which high levels of vitamin A and vitamin E seem to be important in guaranteeing their extreme longevity."[1]

So, exactly what is a free radical? Picture, if you will, an atom that has a nucleus with electrons around it. As electrons circle the nucleus, they are usually paired. When an electron becomes unpaired, it tries to pull an electron from another atom or molecule in order to return to a state of equilibrium. Free radicals are simply atoms with unpaired electrons; they are unstable molecules that damage healthy cells. Free radicals are very aggressive, and as they steal electrons from other atoms, they damage cells in the process. They harm cell membranes and nuclear membranes, and eventually may damage the DNA in the nucleus of the cell. Also, when free radicals steal electrons from other atoms, these atoms become free radicals themselves, leading to a chain reaction. This can create a vicious cycle, leading to damage and destruction of cells and eventually to chronic diseases.

Now free radicals are generated in our bodies simply by breathing. Normal metabolism creates free radicals referred to as reactive oxygen species (ROS). Just as smoke comes from a fire, free radicals come from the normal metabolism and production of energy in the mitochondria of our bodies. Foods—including hydrogenated and partially hydrogenated fats; highly processed foods, sugar, fried foods, and polyunsaturated fats found in salad dressings, cooking oils, sauces, gravies, and so on—also will create excessive free radicals.

Many diseases are inflammatory and are creating tremendous amounts of free radicals, including most cancers, arthritis, coronary artery disease, asthma, Alzheimer's disease, Parkinson's disease, multiple sclerosis, lupus, colitis, and autoimmune diseases. Frequent colds, flu, sinus infections, bronchitis, and bladder and yeast infections create more free radicals. Trauma from sprains, strains, muscle aches, and even excessive exercise creates a tremendous amount of free radicals.

This is why those who overtrain, as well as long-distance runners and marathoners, appear to actually age faster.

And finally, there is our toxic exposure. Unfortunately no one is exempt. There are pesticides and other toxins in our food, water, and air, which create an added burden on the liver. In the detoxification process by the liver, more free radicals are produced, and the toxic burden may be so great that the liver is unable to keep up with detoxification. These toxins increase in the body, which causes the production of more free radicals. Inhaling side stream smoke and car exhaust, drinking tap water with chlorine and all the other chemicals, eating the standard American diet laced with chemicals and inflammatory foods—these all are producing a flood of free radicals that are causing diseases, which create even more free radicals. It becomes a vicious cycle of ever-increasing free radicals. Unfortunately Americans are running to their doctors, who are prescribing medicines that turn off symptoms. Yet these medicines create a greater burden on the liver and cause the production of more free radicals and usually cause nutrient deficiencies.

The answer to free radicals is simple: antioxidants. Antioxidants have the ability to neutralize free radicals. Antioxidants are to free radicals what water is to a raging forest fire burning out of control. Of course, it also involves choosing more living foods, detoxification, and the other pillars of health. But antioxidants are the number one key for the free-radical riddle.

Just think about what happens when you squeeze lemon juice on an exposed slice of apple. The vitamin C and bioflavonoid antioxidants in the lemon quench free radicals, slowing down the oxidation process, which means it takes *much* longer for the apple slice to turn brown. That's why antioxidants are usually added to processed food—to prevent oxygen from combining with different food components. Without them, many processed foods would become stale, rancid, or inedible.

Researchers have known for years that there are literally thousands of different compounds that function as antioxidants. Many are found in foods and supplements, and others are produced by our bodies. That's right, our bodies have developed a powerful army of antioxidants that neutralize free radicals. By consuming living foods containing powerful antioxidants and phytonutrients, taking specific antioxidant supplements, and supporting our own antioxidants produced by our bodies, we will be able to quench many free-radical reactions.

Different antioxidants are able to neutralize free radicals in every part of the body. I believe that it's important to have adequate amounts of three key antioxidants produced by the body and five key antioxidants from supplements. Instead of discussing all the antioxidants, I'll focus on the key antioxidants and a few others.

Key Antioxidants

The key antioxidants that our bodies produce include glutathione, superoxide dismutase (SOD), and catalase.

Glutathione

Glutathione is a 3-amino-acid peptide (or tripeptide) consisting of glycine, glutamine, and cysteine. You may not have heard of this powerful superantioxidant, but in my opinion it is truly the master antioxidant and master detoxifier. When glutathione levels in cells drop too low, cell death occurs.

This is why glutathione is essential to the health of every cell in the body. It helps control inflammation, is critical for the immune system, boosts energy, and protects cells and tissues from free radicals, which protects you from disease.

Furthermore, glutathione is important for optimal function of the five most important organs in the body—the heart, lungs, brain, liver, and kidneys. Glutathione also is required for optimal function of the immune system and for maintaining healthy eyes. Glutathione is considered the most abundant and most important antioxidant in the human body.

It is a powerful antioxidant that is produced in the liver and works throughout the body in cells, tissues, and fluids to detoxify free radicals created from oxygen known as reactive oxygen species (ROS). It simply acts as a powerful detoxifier and free-radical quencher. When one is exposed to a high level of toxins, glutathione is depleted faster than it can be produced, setting the stage for toxin-induced diseases, including cancer. Glutathione can be synthesized from three amino acids: cysteine, glutamic acid, and glycine. It also can be obtained in the diet by consuming fresh fruits and vegetables, cooked fish, and meats.

Cellular Cycle

Ninety to 95 percent of your body's sixty trillion to one hundred trillion cells are replaced every year.

Vitamin C and N-acetyl cysteine (NAC) increase the rate of synthesis of glutathione. I recommend between 500–1,000 mg once or twice a day of NAC. The herb milk thistle helps prevent the depletion of glutathione and actually can raise the level of glutathione in the liver by up to 35 percent. To raise glutathione levels, NAC, vitamin C, and milk thistle are important supplements to consider.[2] Refer to appendix A for information on Cellgevity, which contains RiboCeine, the new glutathione booster that is superior to all others.

Superoxide dismutase (SOD)

SOD is an antioxidant that also works to detoxify the free radical superoxide to hydrogen peroxide, which is also a free radical. SOD then works with another antioxidant, catalase, to break down peroxide to water. It also works with glutathione to inactivate both peroxide and lipid peroxides. SOD is made from three basic minerals: copper, zinc, and manganese. Copper and manganese come from whole grains and nuts, and zinc comes from egg yolks, milk, oatmeal, nuts, legumes, and meat. Supplements of SOD are generally ineffective. Simply taking a good multivitamin that contains adequate amounts of copper, zinc, and manganese usually will help supply adequate amounts of SOD in most non-diseased states. However, in elderly individuals—and especially those with disease—supplementation with copper, zinc, and manganese may not be enough. They probably will need a combination of powerful antioxidant herbs, which increase the production of catalase in the body. These herbs include green tea, turmeric, bacopa, milk thistle, and ashwagandha.

Catalase

Catalase is a powerful antioxidant and is an iron-dependent enzyme. It is designed to prevent a buildup of hydrogen peroxide, another free radical, in the body. Catalase in the skin converts hydrogen peroxide to water. It also oxygenates the epidermis to form smooth, younger skin.

Years ago when I was working on the original edition of my book *Toxic Relief*, I experimented with different types of fasts, including water fasts, juice fasts, and partial fasts. On a seven-day water fast I noticed little white spots forming on my arms and legs. I broke the fast immediately. While it looked like tiny drops of bleach had splashed on my skin, in fact my system had formed a lot of free radicals and hydrogen peroxide. During the fast I had exhausted my catalase, and I did not have enough catalase antioxidant to convert the peroxide to water. I have since noticed many patients with these tiny white spots who have been helped with supplements. SOD and catalase are actually metabolic enzymes that work together and are the body's first line of defense against oxidative stress. Supplements of SOD and catalase, however, are generally ineffective since they are broken down during digestion.

Unfortunately aging is associated with increased levels of free radicals and decreased production of SOD and catalase. However, a unique combination of antioxidant herbs is able to increase production of these powerful antioxidants.[3] Catalase and SOD are referred to as catalytic antioxidants. A catalyst simply promotes a reaction and isn't consumed in the reaction. In other words, these powerful antioxidants can quench millions of free radicals and are not spent in the process, but they can continue to destroy more free radicals at another time. These antioxidant enzymes work inside the cell. The herbs that make up this powerful antioxidant combination include green tea, ashwagandha, turmeric, bacopa, and milk thistle.

Other Antioxidants

Lester Packer, PhD, is a leading researcher in antioxidants and author of the classic 1999 book *The Antioxidant Miracle*[4], his first written for a general readership. Dr. Packer has identified five specific antioxidants that he says are the key antioxidants to protect against heart disease, cancer, Alzheimer's disease, cataracts, and other diseases associated with aging. He believes that the body is best protected by a blend of antioxidants working in synergy with each other. He theorizes that antioxidants are more effective and able to prevent cellular damage when they are present in a balanced combination. Simply put, they work best as a team. He identifies the most important antioxidants as vitamin C, vitamin E, coenzyme Q_{10} (CoQ_{10}), alpha lipoic acid, and glutathione (which I have already discussed). Antioxidants work by protecting different parts of the cell; therefore, a team of antioxidants will provide free-radical protection for the entire cell. Vitamin C protects the water-soluble interior of the cell, and fat-soluble vitamin E protects specific areas of the cell's fatty outer membrane. As I mentioned in chapter 6, there are eight different forms of vitamin E: alpha-, beta-, delta-, and gamma-tocopherol, and alpha-, beta-, delta-, and gamma-tocotrienol. Alpha lipoic acid protects both the inside of the cell and the outside cell membrane.

Most multivitamins will contain vitamin C and only one form of vitamin E (d-alpha-tocopherol). In addition, most individuals are not getting lipoic acid, CoQ_{10}, or glutathione or a supplement that increases glutathione. Avoid the synthetic form of vitamin E that is derived from petroleum. It is called "dl-alpha-tocopherol" or "dl-alpha-tocopheryl."

Lipoic acid

Alpha lipoic acid is a naturally occurring compound that is synthesized by plants and animals, even humans. In its reduced form (R-dihydrolipoic acid, or R-DHLA), it also functions as a powerful antioxidant to protect the liver and help detoxify the body from the effects of medication and radiation. It binds metal ions and prevents them from generating free radicals. It neutralizes free radicals in both the water-soluble and fat-soluble parts of the body. Lipoic acid also helps the body "recycle" and extend the life span of vitamin C, glutathione, CoQ_{10}, and vitamin E. Lipoic acid has been shown to elevate intracellular glutathione levels. It improves insulin metabolism in type 2 diabetes and has been used to treat diabetic neuropathy in Germany for more than twenty years.[5] The R-form alpha lipoic acid is also an excellent form of lipoic acid. The two most powerful forms of lipoic acid are R-DHLA and R-form alpha lipoic acid. I usually recommend alpha lipoic acid 300 mg two times a day.

Coenzyme Q_{10} (CoQ_{10})

The aforementioned CoQ_{10} is a powerful antioxidant that is concentrated in heart cells. It plays a critical role in the production of energy in every cell in the body. It functions as a coenzyme in the energy-producing pathways of every cell in the body and is an important antioxidant that will fight the oxidation that creates free radicals as well as the oxidation of low-density lipoprotein (LDL) and other lipids. CoQ_{10} is found in many foods, such as broccoli, Chinese cabbage, spinach, raw nuts, ocean fish and shellfish, pork, chicken, and beef. However, in a normal diet, we get only 2–5 mg of this important vitamin-like compound, so it is wise to add it in supplement form as well.

CoQ_{10} is one of the best "electron donors" that gives its electrons freely to electron-deficient free radicals, rendering them harmless. It also restores oxidized vitamin E into a useful form. By giving electrons to vitamin E—which, as you recall, is another important antioxidant—it "recycles" vitamin E to get it back into the free-radical fight once again. In this way when supplements of vitamin E and CoQ_{10} are combined, LDL becomes more resistant to oxidation than when you take vitamin E alone. This combination also has been shown to reduce C-reactive protein (CRP) levels in laboratory animals.

Deficiencies are commonly seen in periodontal disease, heart disease, diabetes, HIV, and AIDS. The amount of CoQ_{10} produced by the body declines with age, so I strongly recommend individuals older than fifty use a supplement. However, you should definitely supplement CoQ_{10} if you are taking cholesterol-lowering drugs, such as Mevacor, Pravachol, Lipitor, Crestor, or Zocor. Not all CoQ_{10} is equal. Many forms are synthetic and don't have studies showing that the CoQ_{10} is actually absorbed into the cell. There is also a better form of CoQ_{10} that is actually absorbed into the brain and is able to protect the brain cells.[6] In recent years a reduced form of CoQ_{10} was developed; it is a more powerful antioxidant than regular CoQ_{10}. Realize as many as 30 percent of people may not be able to convert adequate amounts of CoQ_{10} to its active form ubiquinol or reduced CoQ_{10}. CoQ_{10} is found in sardines, spinach, peanuts, and beef. I recommend at least 100 mg of ubiquinol a day or 100 mg of regular CoQ_{10} once a day.

Pyrroloquinoline quinone (PQQ)

PQQ is a coenzyme and antioxidant. It provides defense to the body's cells against free radicals and the damage they cause. However, research has found that not only does it protect cells, but it also actually generates growth of mitochondria. It actually can reverse cellular aging and mitochondrial dysfunction, which is associated with many diseases that come with age. This powerful antioxidant is not one you should overlook.[7] I usually recommend 20 mg once or twice a day.

Chapter 10

PHYTONUTRIENTS: THE RAINBOW OF HEALTH

ANOTHER MAJOR INGREDIENT in achieving an optimal state of health is a class of substances known as phytonutrients (also called phytochemicals). Phytonutrients are biologically active substances that give fruits and vegetables their color, flavor, smell, and natural disease resistance.

They offer major benefits for your body, starting with the key role they play in preventing cancer and heart disease. According to some researchers, forty thousand phytonutrients may one day be cataloged. At the present time there are over two thousand known phytonutrients. These compounds protect plants from pests, excessive amounts of ultraviolet radiation, and disease. Each plant has thousands of different phytonutrients that provide protection from free radicals because they contain natural antioxidants.[1]

In humans phytonutrient consumption is associated with reduced rates of many different cancers. Phytonutrients also protect against heart disease and protect against or slow the progression of dementia and age-related cognitive decline. They increase longevity, are associated with reduced rates of chronic disease, and protect us against cataracts and macular degeneration. Regular consumption of phytonutrients is the best natural health insurance policy that I can recommend for protection from degenerative diseases, including cancer and heart disease.

Phytonutrients work in your body to save you from various threats, including some you likely don't recognize. For example, saponins, found in kidney beans, lentils, chickpeas, and soybeans, may prevent cancer cells from multiplying. A phytonutrient found in tomatoes interferes with the chemical process that creates carcinogens. The list of wonderful things phytonutrients do goes on and on.[2]

The Healing Power of Plants

Approximately two-thirds of all drugs are derived from plants.[3]

According to the most recently published dietary guidelines from 2010, the US Department of Agriculture (USDA) and US Department of Health and Human Services recommend that Americans consume five to thirteen servings of fruits and veggies a day, but most Americans do not consume even the minimum of five servings. In a survey that covered 2007–2010, the Centers for Disease Control and Prevention said that 76 percent of the population didn't meet fruit intake recommendations and 87 percent did not meet vegetable intake recommendations.[4] Unfortunately this means that most Americans are missing out on the great benefits provided by the phytonutrients found in fruits and vegetables.

Healthy Colors

Fruits and vegetables can be grouped according to color. Each group has its own set of phytonutrients that provide unique protective benefits.

Typically phytonutrients are classified by their chemical structures. This is an extensive classification, and it is also quite confusing since many phytonutrients provide similar protection. The main classifications include:

- Organo-sulfurs, such as cruciferous vegetables and the sulfur compound in garlic
- Terpenoids, such as limonene in citrus as well as carotenoids, tocopherols, tocotrienols, etc.
- Flavonoids, including certain red/purple-pigmented fruits and vegetables
- Isoflavonoids and lignans, found in soy foods and flaxseed
- Organic acids, found in whole grains, parsley, licorice, and citrus fruits

Since there are so many different phytonutrients, they are also classified in families, and this depends on the similarities in their structure. As you can see, it can be quite confusing! That's why I like to simply group them by color.

Our goal should be to include as many colors as possible in our daily diet. Approximately half of all Americans don't even eat one piece of fruit all day, and most others will eat the same fruit or vegetable day after day. We need to try and consume all seven colors of the phytonutrient rainbow every day to receive the protection we need. To do this, we need to eat a variety of foods. Eating a colorful salad every day and/or taking a powerful phytonutrient powder are two easy ways to make sure you are consuming all seven phytonutrient color groups.

Think of phytonutrients as a "rainbow of health," God's promise to you to keep you healthy. Let's look at each group.

Red

Tomatoes, watermelon, guava, and red grapefruit contain a powerful carotenoid called *lycopene,* which is about twice as powerful as beta-carotene. Lycopene is the main pigment responsible for the red color. Lycopene is the most abundant carotenoid in the prostate, and high blood levels of lycopene are linked to prevention of heart disease and prostate cancer. A study conducted by Harvard researchers examined the relationship between carotenoids and the risk of prostate cancer. Only the carotenoid lycopene was associated with protection. Men who ate more than ten servings of tomato-based food a week had a 35 percent decreased risk of prostate cancer compared with those eating less than one and a half servings a week. Tomato juice was the one exception; there is no correlation between intake of tomato juice and protection against prostate cancer. Men who consumed at least 6.5 mg a day of lycopene from tomato products specifically were shown to have the highest level of protection against prostate cancer.[5] Men over forty should especially begin eating more organic tomatoes and organic tomato sauce cooked with organic extra-virgin olive oil to get the protection against prostate cancer. About one man in six may develop prostate cancer during his lifetime.[6]

You Say "Tomatoe"; I Say "Tomato"

Did you know that tomatoes are really a fruit and not a vegetable? That's because, botanically speaking, a tomato is the ovary, along with its seed, of a flowering plant—hence, it is a fruit. But back in the late 1800s, when US tariff laws imposed a duty on vegetables but not fruits, the truth about tomatoes was called into question. The US Supreme Court settled this controversy in 1893, declaring that the tomato is a vegetable, along with cucumbers, squashes, beans, and peas, using the popular definition that classifies vegetables by use, that they are generally served with dinner and not dessert. The case is known as *Nix v. Hedden.*[7]

Red/purple

Blueberries, blackberries, hawthorn berries, raspberries, grapes, eggplant, red cabbage, and red wine contain a powerful flavonoid called anthocyanidin, which is the pigment responsible for the brilliant, beautiful red/blue and purple colors. These colors actually draw us to these attractive fruits and vegetables, which in turn protect us from a host of diseases. Anthocyanidins protect cells from free-radical damage in water-soluble and fat-soluble compartments of the body. They have approximately fifty times the antioxidant activity of vitamin C and are twenty times more powerful than vitamin E. They also may help prevent arthritis and atherosclerosis.

Pine bark, grape seeds and skins, bilberry, and cranberry contain another flavonoid called proanthocyanidin, which is a significant source of antioxidants. These powerful phytonutrients—anthocyanidin and proanthocyanidin—strengthen and repair connective tissue and stimulate the synthesis of collagen. They help strengthen capillaries and to maintain elastin, which assists in maintaining the elasticity in our skin and blood vessels, thus aiding in preventing wrinkles, spider veins, and varicose veins.

Resveratrol is found in red grape skins and seeds, purple grape juice, and red wine; it is a phenolic compound that inhibits the development of cancer in animals and also helps prevent the progression of cancer. It decreases the stickiness of platelets, preventing blood clots, and it helps blood vessels remain open and flexible. This powerful phytonutrient also raises the high-density lipoprotein (HDL), or "good," cholesterol.

Strawberries and cranberries also contain powerful flavonoids. There are over four thousand unique flavonoids, but the fruits and vegetables listed above are some of the best sources of them. Flavonoids have anti-inflammatory, anticarcinogenic, antitumor, and antiviral activity. They are powerful antioxidants and metal chelators. They are also important dietary supplements to prevent both cancer and heart disease.

Orange

Orange-colored fruits and vegetables, including carrots, mangos, cantaloupes, pumpkin, sweet potatoes, yams, squash, and apricots, have high amounts of carotenoids. Typically the more orange the fruit or vegetable is, the higher the concentration of provitamin A carotenoids.

There are more than six hundred carotenoids, with about fifty that can be transformed into vitamin A. Orange fruits and vegetables generally are high in beta-carotene.

Lobster and salmon are pink because they have ingested plants containing carotenoids, which has colored their tissues. Even egg yolks get their yellow color from carotenoids eaten by the hen.

Carotenoids quench singlet oxygen, which is a reactive oxygen species (free radical) that damages cells and tissues. They also help prevent cancer and heart disease. The antioxidants vitamin E, vitamin C, lipoic acid, and CoQ_{10} help replenish carotenoids in tissues. The body converts beta-carotene, a carotenoid, into vitamin A as needed. Beta-carotene that is left over is able to quench free-radical reactions and prevents cholesterol from oxidizing, helping to prevent plaque formation in arteries. A diet high in carotenoids, especially alpha-carotene, is protective against cancer.

However, synthetic beta-carotene supplements actually increase the risk of lung cancer in smokers! In one study of twenty-nine thousand men in Finland who smoked and drank alcohol, the men were given beta-carotene (20 mg a day) and/or vitamin E. There was an 18 percent increase in lung cancer in the beta-carotene group.[8]

Beta-carotene used in supplements is mainly the synthetic, trans form. Foods such as carrots supply mixed carotenoids and include the natural forms, which are better than synthetic antioxidants. Instead of taking only beta-carotene, consider organic orange fruits and veggies that have mixed carotenoids, which work together to protect the body. The synthetic beta-carotene supplements may trigger cancer in smokers, and for that reason I recommend orange foods high in carotenoids over beta-carotene supplements.

Orange/yellow

Oranges, tangerines, lemons, limes, yellow grapefruit, papaya, pineapple, and nectarines are rich in vitamin C and citrus bioflavonoids and protect us against free-radical damage since they are powerful antioxidants. Citrus bioflavonoids include rutin, quercetin, hesperidin, and naringin. They are able to increase intracellular levels of vitamin C. Citrus bioflavonoids strengthen blood vessels by supporting the collagen and strengthening the cells that form the inner lining of blood vessels. They also maintain the collagen that forms tendons, cartilage, and ligaments. They prevent the release and production of compounds that promote allergies and inflammation. They have also been used both to prevent and treat bruising, hemorrhoids, varicose veins, and spider veins.

Yellow/green

Spinach, kale, collard greens, mustard greens, turnip greens, romaine lettuce, leeks, and peas are typically rich in lutein and zeaxanthin. *Lutein* is the main carotenoid present in the central portion of the retina of the eye called the *macula*. Lutein is able to reduce the risk of macular degeneration, which is the leading cause of blindness in older adults.

Healthy Veggies

Elderly men who eat lots of dark green and deep yellow vegetables have a 46 percent decrease in heart disease risk compared with men who eat few of these vegetables.[9]

In addition, dark green leafy vegetables contain two pigments, lutein and zeaxanthin, which protect the eye from damage.

A study found that adults with the highest dietary intake of lutein had a

57 percent lower risk of macular degeneration compared with those individuals with the lowest intake. Also, of all the different carotenoids, lutein and zeaxanthin were the most strongly associated with this protection.[10] Lutein also may protect the lens of the eye from sunlight damage, slowing down the development of cataracts. Astaxanthin is another powerful carotenoid found in krill and is one of the most powerful antioxidants known. It accumulates especially in the joints, eyes, and brain, protecting them from free radicals.

Many people don't understand why dark green vegetables are rich in these powerful carotenoids—lutein and zeaxanthin. Carotenoids also occur in dark green leafy vegetables, where their color is concealed by the green pigment called *chlorophyll,* which also protects us against cancer.

Cellular Sickness

When abnormal cells are formed, these cells are designed in a healthy body to undergo programmed cell death, or apoptosis, so that cancer is not formed. Cancer cells do not die but continue to grow and spread due to a mutation in the gene for apoptosis.

Green

Broccoli, cabbage, brussels sprouts, cauliflower, watercress, bok choy, kale, collard greens, and mustard greens are considered cruciferous vegetables. These cancer fighters contain more phytonutrients with anticancer properties than any other family of vegetables. The word *cruciferous* comes from the same word root as *crucifying,* which means "to place one on a cross." The flowers of cruciferous vegetables contain two components that appear similar to the shape of a cross. The powerful cancer-fighting phytonutrients in the cruciferous vegetable family include indoles, isothiocyanates, and sulforaphanes, which are sulfur-containing compounds. They also contain phenols, coumarins, dithiolthiones, and other phytonutrients yet to be discovered. Indoles, including diindolylmethane (DIM) and indole-3-carbinol, are powerful anticancer phytonutrients that are able to suppress cancer growth and induce programmed cell death in a variety of cancers, including breast cancer, prostate cancer, colon cancer, endometrial cancer, and leukemia.[11] They stimulate detoxifying enzymes in the gastrointestinal (GI) tract and the liver. They protect us against carcinogens, which are cancer-causing agents. Indole-3-carbinol supports a healthy estrogen balance and decreases the risk of female-related cancers. Sulforaphanes stimulate liver detoxification enzymes. Isothiocyanates inhibit enzymes that activate carcinogens and stimulate enzymes that remove cancer-causing agents.

Studies have correlated a high intake of cruciferous vegetables, especially cabbage and broccoli sprouts, with lower rates of cancers, especially cancers of the breast, prostate, and colon. Broccoli sprouts have some of the highest concentration of protective phytonutrients. Young broccoli sprouts that are about three days old contain twenty to fifty times more sulforaphane than mature broccoli.

DIM

A powerful phytonutrient was discovered about a decade ago in cruciferous vegetables. DIM, or diindolylmethane, is found in cruciferous vegetables such as broccoli and cauliflower. DIM is vitally important in estrogen balance and may help prevent female-related cancers, such as breast, uterine, ovarian, and cervical dysplasia—a precancerous condition marked by changes in the cells of the cervix.[12]

Eating vegetables only will not supply you with adequate amounts of DIM. You would have to eat about two pounds of broccoli each day to get adequate amounts of DIM. That's why I recommend a supplement.

White/green

Onions and garlic contain powerful phytonutrients. Onions contain the flavonoid quercetin, which has anti-inflammatory properties, antiviral activity, and anticancer properties. Quercetin is often recommended by nutritionists to treat both allergies and asthma. Apples, red wine, and black tea also contain quercetin. In fact, quercetin is the reason why people say, "An apple a day keeps the doctor away." Onions and garlic also contain organic sulfur compounds, which can be used for detoxification by the liver.

Several of the components in garlic have significant anticancer effects. Garlic also inhibits the formation of nitrosamines, which are cancer-causing compounds formed during digestion. Garlic has significant antimicrobial activity against bacteria, viruses, fungi, and even parasites. It also has cholesterol-lowering activities and can even lower blood pressure as well as help prevent blood clots.

POWERFUL PUNCH

Two more powerful phytonutrients that deserve mention are green tea and curcumin.

Green tea's active constituents are polyphenols, including a catechin called epigallocatechin gallate (EGCG). The polyphenols in green tea have been shown to reduce the risk of gastrointestinal cancers, including cancers of the stomach, small intestines, colon, and pancreas, as well as lung and breast cancers. As an antioxidant, green tea is two hundred times more powerful than vitamin E and five hundred times more powerful than vitamin C. It provides powerful antioxidants to help repair damaged DNA. It also activates detoxification enzymes in the liver, which helps defend your body against cancer. The normal amount of green tea consumed by the Japanese is about three cups a day. I recommend organic green tea in dioxin-free tea bags.

Curcumin is the substance that gives turmeric its bright yellow color. Turmeric is the main ingredient of curry powder. It is an herb of the ginger family. Turmeric has significant antioxidant activity, and curcumin is its most powerful component. Both turmeric and curcumin have anticancer effects at all steps of cancer formation. Curcumin has powerful anti-inflammatory properties, especially with acute inflammation such as sprains, muscle strains, and inflamed joints. It also may help individuals with Alzheimer's disease and especially in prevention of Alzheimer's disease by reducing inflammation.[13] It also helps lower cholesterol and prevent blood clots.[14]

Rating the Produce

Another way to judge the benefits of each fruit and vegetable is by each one's oxygen radical absorbance capacity (ORAC). This is a standard tool used by nutritionists to measure foods' antioxidant capacity. The higher the ORAC, the higher the concentration of antioxidants in that food, and the greater protection it provides against free radicals.

In studies of animal and human blood at the Agricultural Research Service's Human Nutrition Research Center on Aging (the chief scientific agency of the US Department of Agriculture), eating plenty of high-ORAC foods "raised the antioxidant power of human blood 10 to 25 percent."[15] Based on these findings, we can see that the first step in raising our antioxidant levels is to increase our intake of high-ORAC foods. Although there is no standard established yet, 3,000–5,000 ORAC units per day from a variety of antioxidant sources is thought to be a good intake level.[16]

A terrific study published in the June 2004 issue of the *Journal of Agriculture and Food Chemistry* tested the antioxidant power of more than one hundred different kinds of fruits, vegetables, nuts, and spices. They came up with a list of the top antioxidant foods. The top twenty are:[17]

1. Mexican red beans (dried)
2. Wild blueberries
3. Red kidney beans
4. Pinto beans
5. Cultivated blueberries
6. Cranberries
7. Artichokes (cooked)
8. Blackberries
9. Prunes
10. Raspberries
11. Strawberries
12. Red Delicious apples
13. Granny Smith apples
14. Pecans
15. Cherries
16. Black plums
17. Russet potatoes (cooked)
18. Black beans (dried)
19. Red plums
20. Gala apples

Blueberries deserve special mention. This colorful fruit contains polyphenols that protect the brain from inflammation and oxidative stress, which in turn may protect the brain from the degenerative effects of aging and from injury from ischemic stroke.[18] Blueberries may even help prevent Alzheimer's disease and Parkinson's disease. When rats suffering from Alzheimer's-like symptoms were supplemented with blueberries in their diets, they were able to perform normally on tests involving memory and motor behavior.[19] I recommend a serving of organic blueberries every day.

The more we learn about phytonutrients and the antioxidants I reviewed in the previous chapter, the more we understand their amazing benefits. There are tens of thousands of them, many yet undiscovered. In addition to eating high-ORAC foods and varied and brightly colored foods, I recommend taking antioxidants and phytonutrients in supplement form since we are usually unable to eat all the colors of the phytonutrient rainbow. Realize that consuming these powerful phytonutrients on a daily basis protects us from developing heart disease, cancer, dementia, macular degeneration, and practically all degenerative diseases.

Chapter 11

THE IMPORTANCE OF HEALTHY FATS

Filmmaker Morgan Spurlock's documentary about his foray into living on McDonald's food secured a "Best Documentary" nomination in the 2005 Academy Awards, after it won that prize at the 2004 Sundance Film Festival, and several others. In 2006 he released *Don't Eat This Book,* which chronicled the full story behind this captivating film. *Super Size Me* chronicled Spurlock's all-McDonald's diet. In just thirty days his weight shot up from 185 to 209 pounds, his cholesterol skyrocketed 65 points, and his body fat jumped from 11 to 18 percent. That's not even including the side effects he suffered, such as mood swings, high blood pressure, and symptoms of addiction.

Check out the nutritional information for McDonald's, and it's easy to see why Spurlock packed on the pounds. A Big Mac checks in at 540 calories, 260 of them from fat, with a total of 28 fat gm (44 percent of daily recommended value), 10 gm of saturated fat, and 960 mg of sodium. The figures for a Quarter Pounder with cheese are nearly identical, except it contains a whopping 1,100 mg of sodium. Increase that Quarter Pounder to a double, and you'll get 780 calories (400 from fat) and 1,310 mg of sodium. Its Bacon Clubhouse burger has 740 calories, 41 gm of fat, and 1,420 mg of sodium.[1]

While Spurlock's plan was an experiment, it symbolized the way millions of Americans live. They derive a significant portion of their calories from fast food and convenience foods that are loaded with fat, sugar, and salt. Because so many treat their bodies this way—by choice—and eat so much unhealthy food that lacks nutritional value, we see the national crisis known as obesity. We are reaping what we sow—not just with obesity, but also its attendant problems, be that heart disease, cancer, hypertension, type 2 diabetes, high cholesterol, reflux disease, or sleep apnea. Such health problems cause a serious loss of quality of life.

Distinguishing Between Fats

Super Size Me can lead you to believe that eating any fat is bad for you. This is simply not true. Overall fats are critically important for our health. Among their many roles, their main purpose in the body is to provide fuel for cells. Each of the trillions of cells in your body is surrounded by a fatty cell membrane composed primarily of polyunsaturated and saturated fats.

The saturated fats provide a rigid support for the cell membrane. The polyunsaturated fats, meanwhile, add flexibility to the cell membranes and allow the transfer of nutrients inside the cells and waste products to be passed outside the cells. These cell membranes need a proper balance of both saturated and polyunsaturated fats.

Likewise, we need a proper balance of fats in our diet to help with the absorption of fat-soluble vitamins, including vitamins A, D, E, and K. We also need fats to produce hormones that regulate inflammation, blood clotting, and muscle contraction. Approximately 60 percent of your brain is composed of fat. You need cholesterol to make brain cells, and most of your cholesterol comes from saturated fats. Fats make up the coverings that surround and protect nerves. They help satisfy hunger for extended periods.

Eating enough of the right kinds of fats is vitally important for good health. The right balance of essential fatty acids keeps the immune system functioning properly and in balance.

The right kinds of fats make all the difference in the world. So, learn to choose good fats and avoid bad ones.

Potentially Bad Fat

The bad fats include the following.

Omega-6 fatty acids

These are found in the following:

- Most commercial salad dressings, sauces, and fried foods
- Sunflower oil
- Safflower oil
- Corn oil
- Sesame oil
- Soybean oil
- Cottonseed oil
- Grape seed oil
- Processed and packaged foods

Americans tend to overconsume omega-6 fatty acids. Omega-6 fatty acids tend to stimulate the body's production of many inflammatory chemicals. That means eating too much of these kinds of fats can increase inflammation. Do not fry foods in omega-6 fats.

Very bad hydrogenated fats

Hydrogenated fats also have a very long shelf life. Yet, these fats tend to take our health from bad to worse, at least when it comes to eating fat. In recent years scientists have learned that partially hydrogenated and hydrogenated fats are far more hazardous to the health than saturated fats, butter, and fatty cuts of meat.[2] In addition, these fats tend to interfere with the body's anti-inflammatory compounds, which, in turn, can increase inflammation and aggravate autoimmune diseases. You can find these fats in the following foods:

- Vegetable shortening
- Margarine and especially hard margarine (These are the worst hydrogenated fats.)
- Most nondairy creamers
- Many salad dressings
- Most baked goods, especially cake icing and donuts
- Many peanut butters
- Most processed foods (These tend to be made with partially hydrogenated fats.)

People with health problems—especially those with heart problems, dementia, memory problems, cancer, or an autoimmune disease—should avoid fried foods. Reject fried chicken, french fries, fried catfish, onion rings, and all other pan-fried or deep-fried foods.

Deep-fried foods are the worst. They contain high amounts of lipid peroxides. These substances actually create free-radical reactions and encourage inflammation. Instead of fried foods, choose baked, broiled, or grilled selections.

Saturated fats

Americans consume too many saturated fats, which are found in fatty cuts of meat, the skin of chicken and turkey, most dairy foods (butter, cheese, cream, ice cream, whole milk), and fatty processed meats.

We have approximately sixty to one hundred trillion cells in our bodies, and every one of them is encased in a cell membrane containing a mixture of unsaturated and saturated fatty acids. These fatty acids provide strength and flexibility. In addition, nutrients are absorbed in the cells through these membranes. Toxins also are released through the cell membranes.

Most individuals with autoimmune diseases eat large amounts of omega-6 fats, fried foods, hydrogenated fats, and saturated fats. These bad fats cause the cell membranes to lose much of their flexibility. When this happens, they cannot absorb nutrients well, properly release toxins, or adequately perform the functions for which they were designed.

Yet limited amounts of saturated fats are important for health. Try to get these fats by eating organically raised free-range meats, chicken, and turkey instead of other meats that are generally high in saturated fats.

GOOD FATS

As I said earlier, good kinds of fats are necessary. You should eat fat every day for the health of your heart, brain, skin, hair, and every part of you.

Monounsaturated fats

Monounsaturated fat is found in extra-virgin or virgin olive oil that is cold-pressed (not heated). You also can get monounsaturated fats in natural organic peanut or almond butter, avocados, olives, macadamia nuts, and especially almonds, walnuts, and hazelnuts. Raw nuts and seeds—not the roasted, salted, flavored, and candied kind—should be a mainstay of your diet. I enjoy almonds, macadamia nuts, and walnuts. Almonds are excellent because they are high in monounsaturated fats and contain about 20 percent protein. Almond butter makes a tasty spread.

If you're new to the use of nuts and seeds as a health measure, go easy with them at first, or you may upset your stomach. Start out light and gradually increase them. As with any food, moderation is the key. Be aware that if you leave nuts unsealed for thirty days, they may become rancid, which will do more harm to you than good. Keep nuts in #1 PETE (polyethylene terephthalate plastic or ceramic) containers, and place them in the refrigerator or freezer until you are ready to use them.

Dan's Famous Salad Dressing

I mentioned earlier that most salad dressings contain omega-6 fatty acids. My brother, Dan Colbert, has a wonderful, healthy recipe for a salad dressing. I like it so much that I wanted to share it with you.

¼ cup balsamic vinegar
2 Tbsp. Frontier's Mama Garlic seasoning mix
1 clove fresh garlic, minced
Juice of one lemon
Pinch of sea salt
2 Tbsp. clean, pure water
⅔ cup organic extra-virgin olive oil

Pour the balsamic vinegar into a glass salad dressing cruet (such as Good Seasons's mixing bottle), add the remaining ingredients in the order listed, and shake to mix. Refrigerate. Makes 1 cup.

TIP: Dressings prepared with olive oil may congeal

when refrigerated. Let the refrigerated dressing reach room temperature before using.

Omega-3 fats

The average American's diet is generally deficient in omega-3 fatty acids. These are the good fats that are vitally important for maintaining a strong and healthy immune system. Omega-3 fatty acids are found in oily, fatty fish (such as salmon, mackerel, herring, and sardines), some marine mammals, algae (seaweed), and flaxseed oil. Scientists believe the best way to obtain adequate omega-3 is direct consumption of docosahexaenoic acid (DHA) and eicosapentaenoic acid (EPA) from fish. DHA protects the brain, reversing signs of brain aging and protecting against development of Alzheimer's and dementia. DHA also plays a role in preventing attention deficit/hyperactivity disorder (ADHD) and impaired learning. EPA protects the heart blood vessels and decreases inflammation. It has anticancer, anti-inflammatory, and antihypertensive effects. EPA reduces the risk of stroke, heart arrhythmias, dementia, and heart attack and lowers triglycerides (fats in the blood).[3]

Alpha-linolenic acid (ALA) is commonly lacking in the standard American diet. The fats in flaxseed, salba seed, hemp seed, chia seed, flaxseed oil, walnuts, and different green vegetables and superfoods are converted in the body into ALA. The body then uses ALA to make EPA and DHA to nourish and protect the heart and brain and to produce a powerful hormone called prostaglandin 3 (PG3), which reduces pain and inflammation and prevents platelets from adhering, which reduces blood clots.

Gamma-linolenic acid (GLA)

GLA is one form of omega-6 fatty acid that is very different from the others. This omega-6 fatty acid works to decrease inflammation. It actually behaves more like an anti-inflammatory omega-3 fatty acid.

GLA is derived from evening primrose oil, borage oil, and black currant seed oil.

The Canola Oil Controversy

The controversy over canola oil, a monounsaturated fat used primarily in cooking and food preparation, illustrates the need to be informed about the differences and nuances of good and bad fat. Although some nutritionists have singled out canola oil as having toxic properties, it is important to understand that the nutritional value of any edible oil can be destroyed and turned into poison, depending on the processing and cooking techniques used. When researchers developed canola oil in the 1970s, they used oil seed from mustard rape (rapeseed). Now canola oil is hybridized to produce an oil with high monounsaturated fat content.

However, controversy remains. Two decades ago, Mary Enig, PhD, one of the top biochemists in the country, found that canola oil had to be partially hydrogenated or refined before it is used commercially.[4] This led to concern over high levels of trans-fatty acids, but canola oil that has not been hydrogenated will not have significant amounts of trans fats. It is important to check the label before purchasing. Also, approximately 90 percent of canola oil is genetically modified, which is usually associated with increased inflammation.

The key to choosing a healthy oil is in the extraction process. Mass market oils are usually chemically extracted from seeds using hexane, a petroleum product that is harmful to the environment and has the potential to leave a residue on the finished product.

Expeller pressing is a much healthier alternative for processing oils. In this process an expeller press crushes seeds with hydraulic action. This process yields less oil than chemical extraction, which is why expeller-pressed oils are usually more expensive. Still, they are the best choice for cooking and eating, and this goes for all oils.

A Word About Fried Foods

Some people resist a call to focus on healthier fats because they don't want to eliminate things they enjoy, such as fried foods. If you still want some fried foods, you can choose to eat healthier by preparing them using organic extra-virgin coconut oil, organic butter, organic ghee (clarified butter), or organic macadamia nut oil, which has a fairly high smoke point—the point at which the oil begins to break down and release free radicals. This may even occur at relatively low temperatures. If you stir-fry with extra-virgin olive oil, do not stir-fry at high temperatures because it has a lower smoke point. Never cook with flaxseed oil.

Avoid frying in polyunsaturated fats (omega-6 fats), such as corn oil, sunflower oil, soybean oil, grape seed oil, or safflower oil. Frying at high temperatures converts these oils to dangerous lipid peroxides, which create tremendous amounts of free radicals. These free radicals can damage the liver and cause chromosomal damage in lab animals. Imagine the amount of damage it is doing in our bodies, and especially in the bodies of our children as we continue to feed them french fries, fried chicken strips, and onion rings.

Most vegetable oils you will find in the supermarket are heat processed. They go through various stages; here is the process in a nutshell. The process begins by taking natural seeds, such as sunflower or sesame, and heating them to about 250 degrees. The seeds are then pressed to expel the oil. Then solvents such as hexane, a petroleum product, are added to dissolve the oil out of the seed or grain, and then heated to 300 degrees to evaporate the solvent. Next begins the degumming process, which removes most of the nutrients from the oil. The oil is left with a yellowish hue after all these processes, so it is then bleached at an even higher temperature and deodorized at temperatures of more than 500 degrees for thirty minutes to one hour. The end result is what you see on the grocery shelf—a clear, odorless oil full of dangerous lipid peroxides. See my book *What Would Jesus Eat?* for more information.[5]

PART III

CLEARING UP THE MISCONCEPTIONS

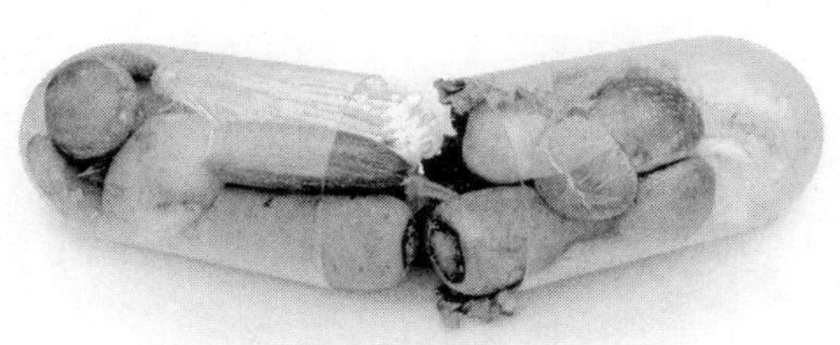

Chapter 12

VITAMIN CONFUSION

If you have ever walked into a health food store, you probably felt the same way many people do: overwhelmed by shelf after shelf crammed with thousands of multivitamins and minerals and individual supplements, each claiming to be the key to your health. Nutritional supplements have become big business, and confusion reigns for the poor consumer.

Supplements are no longer a niche market as they used to be. According to the National Institutes of Health's Office of Dietary Supplements, sales of all dietary supplements totaled $36.7 billion in 2014, including $14.3 billion for all vitamin- and mineral-containing supplements.[1] And yet most chronic diseases continue to rise. For example, in 2011 coronary heart disease, stroke, and other cardiovascular diseases produced about one out of every three deaths in the United States, with 85.6 million Americans living with cardiovascular disease or the after-effects of a stroke.[2] For the years 2009–2011 men in the United States had slightly less than a one in two lifetime risk of developing cancer (meaning the probability of developing or dying from cancer over a lifetime); for women the risk was a little more than one in three.[3] Apparently nutritional supplements are not helping as they should. Why? There are several important reasons.

Disagreement Over Needed Nutrients

There is great confusion among consumers about how much of certain nutrients they need. Some scientists say the human body needs forty essential nutrients; some say fifty. Every decade or so the list of essential nutrients changes, which is why I believe in a conservative approach to supplements. Well-informed scientists disagree about the health benefits of phytonutrients, certain antioxidants, certain vitamins, and so on. Some consider them central to good health; others believe they are peripheral. The list of controversies goes on.

But health experts don't help by creating an alphabet soup of recommended intakes—recommended daily intake (RDI), daily value (DV), daily reference value (DRV), adequate intake (AI), and tolerable upper limit (UL). Few people know what these things mean, how they compare to each other, or how they are measured. And yet people still rely too heavily on the percentages they read on nutrition labels, thinking these percentages represent healthy amounts. In fact, these recommended amounts don't tell you how much you need to be healthy—only how much you need to avoid the most egregious deficiency diseases, such as rickets (caused by lack of vitamin D), beriberi (lack of vitamin B_1), or scurvy (lack of vitamin C). If you get 100 percent of your DV for every nutrient every day, you will avoid these uncommon diseases, but you won't necessarily be healthy. You will have, at best, marginal health, and you will still be exposed to the ravages of degenerative diseases and possibly cancer and heart disease. These recommended daily intakes are often well below the ideal level required for your optimal health.[4]

It's important for consumers to understand that as knowledge of nutrition increases, recommendations change. Nutrients that we now call nonessential may one day be viewed as essential. DVs and RDIs are imperfect but helpful guides. It is each person's job to gain knowledge by reading books such as this one, doing research, and taking charge of their health.

Hidden Hazards

Now that nutritional supplements have become big business, many pharmaceutical companies have jumped on the bandwagon and are manufacturing multivitamins, omega-3 fats (fish oil pills), and many others that are sold in huge quantities at discount stores and supermarkets.

But many companies are more concerned about their profits than your health, and they choose the cheapest option rather than the healthiest one. The evidence is in the pills themselves.

Most mass-produced nutritional supplements contain poor quality synthetic nutrients, which are not nearly as healthy for you as are natural nutrients and may, in fact, be harmful.[5] These man-made multivitamin and mineral supplements usually are made from mineral salts, which are poorly absorbed by your body and therefore vastly less effective but very inexpensive. The manufacturers seem to believe that they can standardize, process, and manufacture vitamins in the same way they manufacture prescription drugs (which, by the way, is not a natural process). The result is an inferior quality of supplements—and usually toxic excipients (fillers) that you didn't expect to make it into your daily tablets.[6] Some big pharmaceutical companies even use ingredients such as toxic partially hydrogenated soybean oil as fillers for their soft gels containing fish oils, vitamin E, and so on. They also add artificial colors, which may have been extracted from coal tar, and put them in their tablets and capsules. A friend of mine calls these "toxic tagalongs."

More than 7 percent of the US population has some sensitivity to these chemicals, so in these cases the supplement is having a dual effect, causing unhealthy side effects while it delivers inferior vitamins and minerals.[7] The larger the tablet, typically the more binding agents and fillers it contains.

Rancid Oils

One of the worst offenders is in fish oil supplements. At my request, many patients come into my office and bring me their fish oil capsules. I stick a needle in and pull out a drop, put it on their finger, and have them taste it. They typically grimace and say, "Why did you make me taste that? It's awful." And yet they swallow those pills daily without thinking about what's inside!

Fish oils and omega-3 supplements can be good for you, but much of the fish oils in supplement form are rancid. Taste it and see for yourself. The fats oxidize quickly and become toxic, causing even more free-radical damage to your body. They do more harm than good. Some fish oils will not even have a rancid odor and taste, yet still contain high amounts of lipid peroxides.[8]

Overall fish oil is an unstable product. The environment, including oxygen and light, begin to oxidize and rancidify fish oil the moment it is extracted from the fish. Fish oil at this late stage of oxidation will smell rancid or fishy. In early stages of oxidation most fish oil products won't smell yet but may still be harmful. Not only that, but also many fish oils aren't tested for polychlorinated biphenyls (PCBs), mercury, or other toxins that can make it into your body through your supplement.[9]

Certain companies add forms of vitamin E and lemon oil, which help keep fish oil from turning rancid.[10] But be aware of what you are taking! While fish oils are very healthy, if you take the wrong ones, you could invite more inflammation and toxins into your body.

If you have been blindly taking supplements on a neighbor's advice or because of something you heard on the radio, it's time to dig deeper and discover what is in that round of pills you consume each day. Supplementation should never be random, but well researched, thought out, and tailored to your specific condition and needs. Otherwise you may be getting things you never wanted in your pills.

Chapter 13

THE DANGERS OF MEGA-DOSING

ONE DAY A man came into my office with a huge suitcase; he even brought it into the exam room.

"What's that?" I asked him.

"These are my supplements," he said as he opened the suitcase to reveal dozens of nutritional supplements, probably worth thousands of dollars. He said he took some for his arthritis, some for high blood pressure, others for diabetes, and still others for digestion problems. Simply the tremendous number of gelatin capsules and fillers that he was taking would give most people digestive problems.

Some people get so excited about taking vitamin supplements that they go overboard and begin mega-dosing. I see it often in my practice. People come in complaining of skin problems, digestion problems, and various other things. It sometimes turns out they are taking too many vitamins, minerals, and other supplements, and they are actually hurting themselves.

This may shock you, but the unhealthiest people I see are the ones who are mega-dosing on supplements. This has to do with their mind-set toward supplements. They have a problem and want to treat the symptoms with a supplement, just as other people treat problems with medications. They are using supplements the way doctors use some drugs—to treat symptoms but not the cause. Sometimes these patients don't want to make other healthy lifestyle and dietary changes, so they rely on pills from the health food store.

But taking pills in high doses can harm you. There is the simple fact that pills are made of much more than the vitamin or mineral or extract you are hoping to consume. These pills often contain all sorts of binding agents, fillers, gels, toxic fats, and dyes.[1] Some of my patients tell me they take hundreds of pills every day. (Granted, they are the exception to the rule, but some literally do this.) They get good deals on supplements at the health food store or through vitamin catalogs, but then they complain to me of fatigue, diarrhea, breakouts, terrible indigestion, belching, and gas. Their supplements have stopped being the cure and are now causing their problems. People sometimes don't produce enough hydrochloric acid in their stomachs and pancreatic enzymes from their pancreas to digest all that gelatin and other fillers in their supplements. Their pills then get passed into their stool because of poor digestion. Mega-dosing also can create sensitivities and allergies to their supplements.

Too Much of a Good Thing

Like anything else in life, too much of a good thing eventually may harm your body. Mega-dosing on one type of vitamin or mineral is no different. For example, mega-doses of vitamin B_6 can lead to peripheral neuropathy or damage to nerves in your arms and legs.[2] And too much vitamin A may promote liver disease.[3] Too much selenium promotes liver impairment,[4] and too much vitamin E is associated with possible heart disease.[5] Taking massive amounts of vitamin C, a fad in past decades, may cause kidney stones.[6] Also, nutrients work synergistically, so simply supplementing with large doses of one vitamin or one mineral may cause imbalances in another vitamin or mineral. For example, a proper balance of copper and zinc is a one-to-ten ratio, and mega-dosing with zinc will dramatically affect that ratio.

The D in Danger

Did you know that taking too much vitamin D can cause the following conditions?

- Nausea
- Constipation
- Weight loss
- Confusion[7]

In the revolutionary *Journal of the American Medical Association* article I cited at the beginning of this book, the authors recommended that all adults take a multivitamin supplement to help prevent chronic disease. Yet they also warned that excessive dosage levels may have toxic effects.[8] One such proof came from the Alpha-Tocopherol, Beta-Carotene Cancer Prevention (ATBC) trial, which tried to determine the long-term effects from vitamin supplements in smokers. The researchers followed the participants for an additional eight years after the trial ended to ensure the accuracy of their results. The study tested the effects of alpha-tocopherol (a form of vitamin E) and beta-carotene on cancer prevention.[9]

The ATBC study concluded that men who smoked and took beta-carotene had an 18 percent greater incidence of lung cancer and an 8 percent increased overall mortality rate. They hypothesized that excessive beta-carotene was somehow worsening the lung cell proliferation induced by smoke. Participants taking vitamin E had 32 percent fewer cases of prostate cancer and 41 percent fewer deaths from prostate cancer, but the risk of death from hemorrhagic stroke increased by 50 percent in men taking alpha-tocopherol supplements. The increase occurred primarily among men with high blood pressure.[10] This information shows that if you have a specific disease such as hypertension or lung cancer, mega-dosing on supplements can actually kill you.

Supplements Are Supplements

Supplements do not exist to replace a healthy diet; they exist to complement it. Taking supplements in high doses or taking an excessive amount of supplements can actually harm you. Generally the unhealthiest patients that I see are the ones who are mega-dosing. If you have been following this pattern, take a break from your supplements for one to two weeks and then one day a week take a break from your supplements, or a supplement sabbath. The results may surprise you.

If you are taking high doses of any single vitamin, mineral, or supplement, or high doses of a combination of these, you may be putting yourself in harm's way. You must stop what you are doing and change your mind-set toward supplements. They are not a cure-all. When it comes to supplements, more is not necessarily better. You must remember that supplements are just that—to supplement a healthy diet. They are not the diet itself. As long as you eat a healthy diet, you don't have to meet all your nutritional needs with supplements. Pills should not be your first source of nutrition; a healthy diet is your foundation. Please refer to my book *Let Food Be Your Medicine*. Supplements are simply to complement your diet to ensure you receive adequate vitamins, minerals, antioxidants, and phytonutrients.

When one of my patients is mega-dosing, I often have him (or her) take a one- or two-week break from supplements. After a week or two with no supplements, the symptoms often go away. After that I may suggest one or two days a week without any supplements. For men, I generally limit supplements to a good whole-food multivitamin, vitamin D_3, an antioxidant, such as CoQ_{10}, a phytonutrient powder, omega-3 supplement, a probiotic, and perhaps a digestive enzyme. For women, I advise the same plan, although sometimes with extra calcium and magnesium.

In your zeal for health, don't mega-dose. Don't treat supplements like drugs or medications. Rather, learn to choose the healthiest kinds of supplements, and avoid impostors. I'll give you advice on this topic in the next chapter.

Chapter 14

HOW TO PICK THE RIGHT SUPPLEMENT

WHAT CONSTITUTES A good multivitamin? The answer is the same things that make living food healthy. Most multivitamins are made of synthetic ingredients and toxic fillers. They may have all the vitamins you need, but the vitamins are typically in suboptimal amounts and in a cheap form made of mineral salts, which are poorly absorbed in an inactive form of the vitamin. The vitamin B_{12} that most use is the inactive form or cyanocobalamin instead of the active form of methylcobalamin. People who take these pills usually don't get the nutrition they need.

These chemical-based supplements also lack that vital combination of nutrients that characterize living foods. Nature never produces nutrients in isolation. Oranges, for example, contain much more than vitamin C. Carrots contain much more than beta-carotene. When you eat them, you get a myriad of vitamins, phytonutrients, flavonoids, and more that interact in ways that are not fully understood, but that we recognize to be healthy.

Substandard Vitamins

Most multivitamins contain cheap mineral salts instead of chelated minerals. Chelated minerals are minerals attached to amino acids, which improve the absorption of minerals.

When you isolate one of these nutrients and take it in high doses, especially in synthetic form, your body may treat it as a foreign substance, and why not? When you only consume synthetic vitamins, there is generally no synergy or balance. It's similar to taking a drug or medication. It ignores the complexity of nutrition.

For example, in recent years pharmaceutical companies jumped on the phytonutrients bandwagon, realizing that these have a certain appeal to consumers. But the manufacturers usually strip out a single phytonutrient and put it into capsules and supplements. The problem is that phytonutrients almost certainly were not meant to be consumed one at a time. There is not a single fruit or vegetable in the world that contains only one kind of phytonutrient, vitamin, or mineral. Nutrients can be isolated, but I am not sure if it will have a healthy effect when it is taken in high doses. Rather, the healthiest supplements combine the enzymes, coenzymes, trace elements, antioxidants, activators, phytonutrients, vitamins and minerals, and many other elements, which all work together synergistically. These supplements are called whole-food supplements and are generally what I recommend.

Nutritionist Paavo Airola, MD, PhD, in his book *How to Get Well*, stated, "When you take natural vitamins, as for instance in the form of rose hips, brewer's yeast, or vegetable oil, you are getting all the vitamins and vitamin-like factors that naturally occur in these foods—that is, all those that are already discovered as well as those that are not discovered yet."[1] In other words, whole-food vitamins are able to provide nutritional balance and synergy, whereas synthetic vitamins typically do not.

Wise Choice

I may recommend supplementation with both pancreatic enzymes and/or hydrochloric acid (HCL), especially for patients over sixty years of age. I prefer that nutritional supplements that are in vegetable capsules are excipient (filler) free and are nonirradiated.

Whole-food supplements combine portions of the plants we know are healthy and those portions we have not yet discovered to be healthy. I believe it's wise to do this because medical knowledge is expanding so quickly that it gets outdated practically every few years. A nutrient we hadn't heard of a year ago can suddenly be discovered to protect against certain kinds of cancer or disease.

You need a comprehensive multivitamin made from living ingredients and combined with living nutrition.

How to Choose a Supplement

The reason we have so many vitamin and mineral deficiencies is because most Americans have embraced fast foods and processed foods, rarely consuming adequate amounts of whole grains, fresh fruits, vegetables, and nuts and seeds, which are excellent sources of these nutrients. (For more information, read my book *Let Food Be Your Medicine*.) So we do need supplements, preferably whole-food supplements.

However, my goal is to simplify your life, not complicate it. When choosing a supplement, you should look for a multivitamin that contains all thirteen vitamins and seventeen to twenty-two minerals with 100 percent of daily values. Also, you need omega-3 fats, a phytonutrient powder, a probiotic, and maybe certain antioxidants, such as CoQ_{10}. *That's it!*

To see what the daily values are according to your age and sex, refer to chapter 8 on minerals. Realize if you consume a healthy diet, you probably will get at least 50 percent of the daily values of vitamins and minerals.

If you are over sixty years of age, you may need extra antioxidants, calcium, vitamin D, sublingual B_{12}, and maybe digestive enzymes. If you already have a disease or simply want more protection, start taking extra antioxidants after the age of forty.

Basics for everyone

When choosing a supplement, here is what I recommend for everyone, regardless of age:

1. Choose a comprehensive multivitamin that has at least 100 percent of the daily value (DV) or recommended daily intake (RDI). (See the chart below.) Start slowly because they may upset your stomach. Start with half the recommended amount and space them out during the day after meals usually twice a day. You may increase the amount as tolerated.

COMPONENTS OF A COMPREHENSIVE MULTIVITAMIN	
Vitamins	Vitamin A, vitamin B_1 (thiamine), vitamin B_2 (riboflavin), vitamin B_3 (niacin), vitamin B_5 (pantothenic acid), vitamin B_6 (pyridoxine), vitamin B_{12}, biotin, folic acid, vitamin C, vitamin D, vitamin E, vitamin K
Minerals	Boron, calcium, chromium, cobalt, copper, iodine, iron, magnesium, manganese, molybdenum, phosphorus, potassium, selenium, silicon, sodium, sulfur, vanadium, zinc

2. Choose a high-quality omega-3 fat to take daily. Start slowly with one a day, and increase as tolerated.

3. Choose a probiotic beneficial bacteria and take it upon awakening. I combine my probiotic with one tablespoon of chia seeds upon awakening.

4. Choose a phytonutrient powder. This powder should contain a combination of colorful organic fruits and vegetables, such as red, yellow, green, orange, and purple. Start slowly with just a teaspoon a day, and increase the amount as tolerated and take one day off each week.

5. Take extra vitamin B_3 at least 1,000–2,000 IU a day.

Supplements in a vegetable-based capsule are far less likely to contain toxic components. Some gelatin capsules are made from animal by-products, and with the concern over mad cow disease in recent years, it's best, if possible, to make sure the supplement is in a vegetable-based capsule made from herbal and vegetable concentrates.

For those fifty and older

If you are fifty years of age or older, you should take a multivitamin, a phytonutrient powder, and omega-3 fats; also make sure you get extra antioxidants, calcium, vitamin D, and a probiotic. (See appendix A for recommended products.)

1. Vitamin E (mixed tocopherols and tocotrienols), 200–400 IU a day (may be present in a multivitamin). Be careful not to take over 400 IU of vitamin E a day.
2. Vitamin C, 250 mg twice a day (may be present in a multivitamin)
3. Coenzyme Q_{10} or ubiquinol (active form of CoQ_{10}) one capsule (100 mg), once a day
4. Alpha lipoic acid, 300 mg two times a day
5. N-acetyl cysteine (NAC), 500 mg twice a day, or MaxOne (RiboCeine), one capsule twice a day
6. Turmeric or curcumin, 500 mg once or twice a day
7. Calcium and vitamin D: calcium, 200 mg three times a day, and vitamin D, 1,000 IU or higher a day. Men generally only need 200 mg of calcium once or twice a day.

For those sixty and older

I recommend a sublingual methyl B_{12} supplement for patients over sixty years of age. After age sixty many Americans do not produce adequate amounts of hydrochloric acid (HCL), which is required for binding B_{12} to intrinsic factor for absorption in the ileum, which is the last part of the small intestines.[2] Follow my recommendations for fifty and older and add the following:

1. Digestive enzymes and/or hydrochloric acid (HCL), one after each meal
2. Sublingual methyl B_{12}, 100 mcg a day

The Importance of Omega-3 Fats

Although I discussed healthy fats in chapter 11, it is worth mentioning again that high-quality fish oils, or omega-3 fats, are vitally important for good health. Realize that many deadly degenerative diseases are inflammatory, such as cancer, heart disease, Alzheimer's disease, arthritis, autoimmune disease, and so on. Fish oil is able to decrease inflammation significantly. I believe omega-3 fats are special fats the body needs as much as it needs vitamins. Much of the research on these powerful fats was done in the 1980s after realizing the Inuit Indians rarely developed heart attacks or rheumatoid arthritis. Yet their diet contained an enormous amount of fat from fish, seals, and whales, which are all high in omega-3 fats.

By decreasing inflammation, fish oil is able to help treat and prevent conditions such as cancer, heart disease, rheumatoid arthritis, psoriasis, migraine headaches, allergies, Alzheimer's disease, and even diabetes. Fish oil also helps balance and stabilize neurotransmitters in the brain, which may be helpful in patients with attention deficit disorder, depression, and bipolar disorder.

Phytonutrients

I discussed the role of these powerful plant pigments in chapter 10, but much of that content centered on the phytonutrients contained in healthy, colorful foods. However, I also believe that *everyone* needs these supplements on a daily basis since multivitamins simply do not provide them. Unfortunately most of us, as well as our children, also are falling way short of the USDA-recommended servings of fruits and vegetables each day. As a result we are falling prey to disease. To get adequate amounts, I recommend a phytonutrient powder, one that provides a combination of colorful organic fruits and vegetables, such as red, yellow, green, orange, and purple, as well as fiber in order to have phytonutrient protection on a daily basis.

Living in Divine Health

Opinions will always differ on what vitamins and minerals to take and on the amounts necessary. Before making any dramatic changes in the amount of vitamins or minerals you add to your daily diet, always consult your personal physician. There are other nutritional supplements that are important, including pomegranate extract, glucosamine sulfate, pyrroloquinoline quinone (PQQ), and supplements for prostate health. However, the ones I have reviewed form the *foundation* for good health. Also, natural, bioidentical hormone replacement therapy is extremely important for women and men, especially over the age of fifty. Refer to appendix A for guidance on how to find physicians who are trained in bioidentical hormone replacement in your area.

Step Into Good Health

Everyone needs a good multivitamin and a phytonutrient supplement. Most everyone needs essential fats in the form of high-grade fish oil and a probiotic. If you are under fifty years of age, start to take a good, whole-food multivitamin, a phytonutrient powder, a probiotic, and an omega-3 supplement. If you are over fifty years of age, you may also need extra antioxidants, calcium, and vitamin D_3.

As more research is done on nutritional supplements, we will find that some supplements may be healthier than we thought and others may be less healthy. It is impossible to banish all confusion regarding supplements, so we must do the best we can with the information we are given for the moment. See appendix A for recommended products.

PART IV

AN A-TO-Z GUIDE

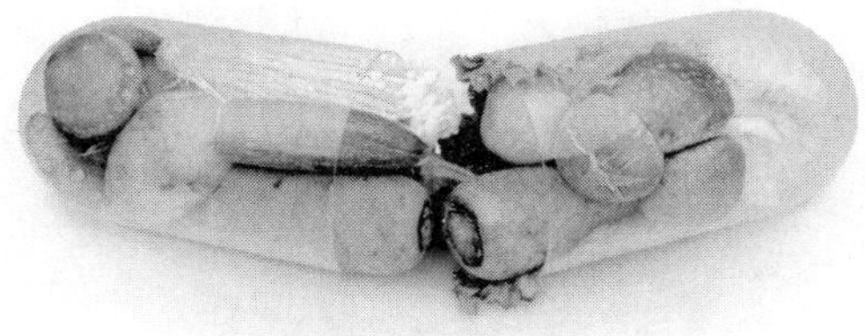

Consult your physician before beginning a supplementation program or if you have any qustions about your health.

Chapter 15

FROM ADD/ADHD TO THYROID DISORDERS

ADD/ADHD

VITAMINS AND MINERALS are uniquely programmed to keep your child's mind and body functioning properly. Today's fast-food lifestyles make it tough for your child to get all the nutrients he needs. For those with attention deficit disorder or attention deficit/hyperactivity disorder (ADD/ADHD), I typically check a neuroscience test that checks brain neurotransmitters and balances them with amino acids and nutrients. I also check an antigen leukocyte cellular antibody test (ALCAT) to identify food sensitivities and foods that trigger their symptoms. In addition, you can provide powerfully beneficial supplements that will directly impact your child's ability to focus and process information. Let's take a look at a powerful brain-boosting program of vitamins, minerals, nutrients, and other supplements that can change your youngster's life forever. Refer to *The Bible Cure for ADD and Hyperactivity* and *Let Food Be Your Medicine,* and follow the dietary program for ADD/ADHD.

Vital vitamins and minerals

I recommend glutathione-boosting supplements for ADD/ADHD, such as N-acetyl cysteine (NAC) 250–500 mg two times a day or MaxOne one or two times a day as well as pyrroloquinoline quinone (PQQ), 10–20 mg one or two times per day, and ubiquinol, which is the active form of coenzyme Q_{10} (CoQ_{10}), 100 mg one or two times per day. In addition, I recommend the following supplements.

Multivitamin/multimineral

Start your child on a good comprehensive multivitamin and mineral formula that supplies the required daily allowances of vitamins and minerals. It should be taken daily. Children eight years old and older can usually swallow a whole-food multivitamin and mineral in capsule form. If a child cannot swallow a capsule, a chewable or liquid multivitamin may be used. It is, however, very difficult to get adequate vitamins and minerals in chewable or liquid multivitamins. Therefore, I recommend that parents open the contents of a whole-food vitamin capsule and sprinkle it in applesauce and give it to their child one to two times a day. See appendix A for more information.

Zinc

Children often have zinc deficiencies because the main sources for zinc include foods that many children don't like—foods such as eggs, seafood, nuts, seeds, and whole-grain bread. Zinc deficiencies affect both learning and behavior. Check to be sure that your multivitamin contains zinc. Children from seven months to three years should receive 3 mg of zinc per day. Children aged four through eight should receive 5 mg per day, and children nine through thirteen should receive 8 mg per day.[1] This is found in most multivitamins.

B-complex vitamins

Your child's behavior and ability to learn also can be affected when B-complex vitamins are lacking in his diet. A good multivitamin also will contain B-complex vitamins. Some children with ADD/ADHD have a mutation in their methylenetetrahydrofolate reductase (MTHFR) gene, and require the active form of folic acid. Ask your pediatrician to do a MTHFR Thermolabile Variant DNA Analysis.

Iron

Most American children aren't getting enough iron in their diets. Without enough iron, your child's attention span can be decreased. Adolescent girls are especially vulnerable to deficiencies in iron.

A simple blood test can determine if your child needs iron. Ask your family physician or pediatrician to test your child for iron deficiency, especially if your youngster has been diagnosed with ADD and ADHD.

Phosphatidylcholine (PC)

The brain-boosting nutrient choline has been proved to be extremely safe for children with ADD. Acetylcholine is an incredible neurotransmitter and is the main brain chemical for thought and memory. You can purchase choline or phosphatidylcholine from any health food store. I also recommend phosphatidylserine (a relative of PC), usually 50–100 mg twice a day with acetyl L-carnitine 250–500 mg two times a day, which usually helps them focus better.

Take 2,000–3,000 mg of phosphatidylcholine two to three times a day. Children under twelve years of age usually need only half this amount, or about 1,000–1,500 mg, two to three times a day.

Acetyl L-carnitine (ALC)

Acetyl L-carnitine (ALC) is a special form of carnitine that aids mental functioning. ALC increases energy across the brain's mitochondrial membrane, and it improves communication between the brain's two hemispheres.

Vitamin B_5

Children twelve and older usually need at least 100 mg of B_5 per day, and children under twelve need approximately 50 mg of B_5 per day. B_5 is very safe. Again, it is best to take this two times a day instead of taking it all at once.

B-complex, which includes all eight B vitamins, vitamin C, and magnesium can all be taken in a comprehensive multivitamin and mineral capsule or tablet.

Fish oil

I recommend docosahexaenoic acid (DHA) supplements (from fish oil or from algae) in gel capsule form with added vitamin E (d-alpha-tocopherol) to prevent rancidity. Fish oil capsules should contain at least 120 mg of DHA. Take one capsule two or three times a day with meals. Some children also benefit from a combination of DHA and EPA. (See appendix A.)

Caution: amino acids and children

Don't place your children on amino acids, even though they can be purchased at a health food store. Phenylalanine and tyrosine are amino acids that are converted to the neurotransmitter norepinephrine, which may help to focus. However, it is important to be under the care of a nutritional doctor to monitor these supplements.

Adrenal Fatigue

Chronic stress, pain, illness, and injury, as well as anxiety and depression, eventually can take a toll on your adrenal glands. These two thumb-sized glands sit atop your kidneys, which manufacture stress hormones. When a stressor or stressors persist, these glands are unable to keep up with the production demands of the body, resulting in adrenal fatigue.

For people suffering from adrenal fatigue, I recommend the following supplements.

De-Stress Formula (DSF)

Many individuals with autoimmune disease have low adrenal function. Therefore, I generally place most of my patients on an adrenal glandular formula, such as DSF, to help support and stabilize the body's stress hormones. The majority of my patients with autoimmune disease benefit from adrenal glandular supplements.

Adrenal glandular supplements contain protomorphogens or extracts of tissues from the adrenal glands of pigs or cattle. These can be taken orally to support human adrenal function. Each organ of the body has a unique mix of vitamins, minerals, and hormones. Glandular substances in pigs and cattle have an "adrenal mix" close to that of the human adrenal glands. Some doctors of natural medicine have used adrenal glandular supplements with their patients for decades and report very positive results.

Take one to two tablets of DSF twice a day, in the morning and at lunch, to supply raw materials to help restore the adrenal function. Occasionally I have to place a patient on three tablets twice a day. Some patients may need to chew the tablet if they are not improving, even though it doesn't taste good. Other good adrenal supplements include Drenamin from Standard Process and Adrenal Support from Gaia Herbs.

Fun Isn't Frivolous

Modern life has more than its share of stress, whether that is too many deadlines, too much to do, a lack of free time... you can name the stresses that fill your life. That's why experts say that having fun isn't a dirty word. They recommend doing something you did as a child, such as playing with an electric train or playing at the park with your grandchildren.

Pantothenic acid (B_5)

Pantothenic acid is known as the "antistress" vitamin because it plays such a vital role in the production of adrenal hormones. Pantothenic acid provides critical support for the adrenal glands as it responds to stress, and adequate supplementation is very important for the health of adrenal glands in most people. I believe vitamin B_5 is the most important B vitamin for restoring and maintaining adrenal function. I typically place patients with adrenal fatigue on 500 mg two times a day.

Vitamin C

Vitamin C is an extremely important vitamin and antioxidant in the battle against stress. The adrenal glands use more vitamin C per gram of tissue weight than any other organ or tissue in the body.

Vitamin C is an antioxidant, and as such it has indirect benefits related to stress. Antioxidants are compounds that help protect the cells from free-radical damage. They are able to disarm free radicals. Antioxidants work synergistically, or as a "team," in the body. For example, vitamin C helps restore vitamin E to its full potency.

The current recommended daily intake (RDI) for vitamin C is 75–90 mg a day to prevent disease.[2] I recommend 250–500 mg two times a day for optimal daily intake. As a water-soluble vitamin, any vitamin C that is consumed and isn't needed by the body will be flushed out through the bloodstream and kidneys.

Medications such as aspirin and oral contraceptives deplete vitamin C in the body. People who develop kidney stones or are on numerous medications should consult their physician about taking additional vitamin C.

Phosphatidylserine

Phosphatidylserine (PS) is an essential component in every cell membrane in the body. I have found that a significant number of patients with adrenal fatigue or low adrenal function have elevated nighttime cortisol levels, which aggravates insomnia. I usually start them on 200 mg of PS in the evening and gradually increase the dose until nighttime cortisol levels are normal.

The average dose of PS is 100 mg in capsule form, and compared with many supplements, PS is quite expensive. Those who are undergoing significant physical stress—such as competitive weight lifters, marathon runners, and others who have elevated nighttime cortisol levels—may find the cost well worth the results. If salivary cortisol levels are elevated in the evening, you may benefit from taking 100–800 mg in the evening or at bedtime.

Adaptogens

An adaptogen is a substance that will help the body adapt to stress by balancing the adrenal gland's response to stress. The end result is that cortisol levels will be neither too high nor too low but will be balanced. One I recommend is *Rhodiola rosea*, an herb native to the mountainous regions of Asia, parts of Europe, and the Arctic. I recommend a product that uses a standardization of 2–3 percent rosavin, the active ingredient of *Rhodiola* used in clinical studies. The common dose is 200–600 mg three times a day.

Others that can help you deal with stress are ginseng, Korean ginseng (take 200 mg one to three times a day, three weeks on and two weeks off), Siberian ginseng, ashwagandha (3–6 gm a day), and magnolia bark. (See appendix A.)

Magnesium

Low magnesium levels are very common in individuals with adrenal fatigue. Approximately 50 percent of the US population is deficient in magnesium.[3] Increased stress as well as adrenal fatigue cause our bodies to have an increased need for magnesium. Magnesium is involved in the activation of more than three hundred enzymes in the body. It is vital to health. When cortisol and adrenaline levels are elevated, there is also an increase of urinary excretion of magnesium. This indicates that in times of stress, our bodies have an increased need for magnesium. The dietary recommendation for magnesium is 300 mg. I commonly recommend 200 mg of magnesium two times a day.

Dehydroepiandrosterone (DHEA)

DHEA is involved in many processes in the human body. It promotes the growth and repair of protein tissue, especially muscle, and it acts to regulate cortisol, negating many of the harmful effects of ongoing excessive cortisol.

When demands for cortisol are increased for a prolonged time, DHEA levels decline and the DHEA no longer is able to balance the negative effects of excess cortisol. A depressed level of DHEA may serve as an early warning sign of adrenal exhaustion.

I recommend either 7-keto DHEA or DHEA in a dose of approximately 50 mg a day for men or 25 mg a day for women. Some DHEA is converted to estrogen. However, 7-keto DHEA does not convert to estrogen.

Pregnenolone

If DHEA is considered the "mother" hormone, then pregnenolone is the "grandmother" hormone. It is a natural hormone discovered in the 1940s and is made largely from cholesterol, which is used, in turn, to make DHEA. When the body is under stress, pregnenolone is used to produce more cortisol.

Pregnenolone is known as the "hormone balancer" since it has the ability to increase levels of steroid hormones that are deficient in the body and can decrease excessive levels of circulating hormones.

Progesterone (for women)

As women age, the ovaries gradually produce less and less progesterone, and eventually the production ceases around menopause. In even younger women suffering from severe adrenal fatigue, cortisol levels are typically low, as are progesterone levels. This is because the body robs progesterone from the ovaries to produce cortisol, which becomes depleted under long-term stress.

Some women benefit from bioidentical progesterone supplementation using transdermal creams or an oral dose of progesterone at bedtime if the patient has insomnia. If women have low progesterone levels, I recommend a bioidentical progesterone cream. One can purchase this at a health-food store or see a doctor for a prescription. However, I do not recommend synthetic progesterone.

Anxiety and Depression

There are wonderful natural substances that can help you overcome depression and anxiety: vitamins, minerals, amino acids, and herbs. These powerful substances are readily available in health food stores. Although they are no substitute for consulting a physician or professional counseling, they will usually help you overcome depression. Please refer to my books *The New Bible Cure for Depression and Anxiety* and *Let Food Be Your Medicine* for a dietary program for anxiety and depression.

Nutrient deficiencies and supplements

Two specific nutrient deficiencies have been associated with depression and anxiety: the B vitamins and magnesium. I believe that in order to alleviate both depression and anxiety, it is important to take a good comprehensive multivitamin that contains the B vitamins and magnesium that will enable your body to make the necessary neurotransmitters, or "feel good chemicals," to begin to change your mood. A comprehensive multivitamin and omega-3 fatty acid supplement, along with a healthy diet, provide the foundation for changing your mood.

Let me discuss these nutrients briefly and then give you my specific recommendations for supplements.

The B vitamin family

As I mentioned in chapter 7, there are eight essential B vitamins, and these are important in patients who have depression and anxiety. Vitamin B_6 is extremely important in patients with depression and anxiety because it is critical to the synthesis of the neurotransmitters serotonin and dopamine. Elevated levels of the amino acid homocysteine increase the risk of depression. However, three B vitamins—B_6, B_{12}, and folic acid—generally lower the homocysteine levels. These B vitamins also function as "methyl donors," which are absolutely necessary for human neurotransmitters to function efficiently.

Many patients with depression have a malfunction in the methylenetetrahydrofolate reductase (MTHFR) gene and are unable to convert folic acid to the active form of folic acid, which is methyltetrahydrofolate (MTHF). These patients usually will notice significant improvement in their symptoms of depression when they take MTHF. In fact, a new medicine for depression is Deplin or MTHF. I usually will place them on MTHF 5–15 mg a day. If you are depressed ask your doctor to check the MTHFR Thermolabile Variant, DNA analysis. Deplin is a rather new medicine but is really the active form of folic acid (L-methyl folate). It comes in 7.5 mg and 15 mg and is used especially in patients with major depressive disorder as adjunctive support for patients on an antidepressant.[4]

Researchers have found that depressed patients are commonly deficient in B_6, B_{12}, and folic acid. I have found that vitamin B_6 levels are especially low in women on birth control pills. To ensure you have adequate amounts of B_6, as well as the other important B vitamins, take approximately 800 mcg of folic acid, 500 mcg of B_{12}, and 2–10 mg of B_6. Good comprehensive multivitamins will contain adequate amounts of these important B vitamins.

- **Magnesium**

Magnesium is very important for more than three hundred enzymatic reactions in the body. Magnesium may help reduce nervousness and anxiety and may help you sleep, especially if it is taken at bedtime. It also helps prevent muscle spasms, heart attacks, and restless legs syndrome, and it relaxes muscles. If you suffer from muscle spasms, eye twitches, jittery feelings, and anxiety, it is highly likely that you are not taking sufficient amounts of magnesium.

I typically recommend approximately 300–400 mg of magnesium a day; higher doses than this may cause diarrhea. Good comprehensive multivitamins will usually contain adequate amounts of magnesium. For patients with insomnia, it's best to take magnesium at bedtime.

Supplements for depression

Use these supplements for depression specifically.

S-adenosyl methionine (SAM-e)

This is the natural form of the amino acid methionine that has been sold as an antidepressant medication in Europe for more than twenty years. SAM-e not only works as an antidepressant with few or no side effects, but it also may improve cognitive function and is useful in treating osteoarthritis as well as liver disease.

Numerous studies have shown the efficacy of SAM-e in treating the symptoms of depression. SAM-e actually helps raise the neurotransmitters serotonin, dopamine, and norepinephrine in the brain.

Many physicians, especially in Europe, believe that SAM-e is just as effective as standard antidepressant drugs in treating depression. In fact, in 2003, after the US Department of Health and Human Services reviewed one hundred clinical trials on SAM-e, it concluded that SAM-e works as well as many prescription medications without the side effects.[5]

SAM-e must be taken on an empty stomach. I usually recommend starting on low doses of 200 mg twice a day on an empty stomach, and gradually working up to 400–800 mg twice a day on an empty stomach, usually about thirty minutes before meals.

This supplement is somewhat expensive. Please take a multivitamin with adequate amounts of B_6, B_{12}, and folic acid to avoid elevated levels of the toxic amino acid homocysteine.

5-hydroxytryptophan (5-HTP) and L-tryptophan

The amino acid called 5-hydroxytryptophan (5-HTP) was discovered in the 1990s and is derived from the seed of the *Griffonia simplicifolia* plant from Africa. Its processing does not involve fermentation, and the seed is a natural source. When the amino acid L-tryptophan combines with vitamin C, 5-hydroxytryptophan is produced in the body.

L-tryptophan and 5-HTP help restore the levels of the important neurotransmitter serotonin, which helps alleviate depression and anxiety by regulating mood, behavior, appetite, and sleep.

There are several reasons I feel 5-HTP is superior to L-tryptophan.

Researchers have found that in clinical trials, approximately 70 percent of 5-HTP administered orally is absorbed directly into the bloodstream.[6] This means that 5-HTP tends to be absorbed better than L-tryptophan. This also means that it is not necessary to take as high a dose of 5-HTP as L-tryptophan since more of it is delivered to the brain.

L-tryptophan and 5-HTP are also quite effective in treating depression, which is usually associated with low serotonin levels. The normal dose of 5-HTP is 50 mg three times a day with meals or 150 mg at bedtime. However, after a few weeks you may increase the dose to 100 mg three times a day with meals or 300 mg at bedtime. You should not take 5-HTP with any other antidepressants, such as Prozac, Zoloft, and Paxil.

L-tryptophan usually comes in a 500-mg dose. I usually recommend taking two to three capsules at bedtime. I recommend USP pharmaceutical grade, especially with L-tryptophan since the Centers for Disease Control and Prevention (CDC) linked a contaminated batch of L-tryptophan to a rare blood disorder called eosinophilia-myalgia syndrome (EMS), which was responsible for multiple deaths in 1989. It was taken off the market for a while but has since been reapproved for use. Do not take both L-tryptophan and 5-HTP except under the supervision of a physician. It usually takes about three to four weeks to feel the benefits of these powerful amino acids.

L-tyrosine

This is an amino acid that is eventually converted to dopamine, norepinephrine, and epinephrine, which are neurotransmitters. Over the years I have found that higher doses of L-tyrosine are fairly effective in treating some cases of depression.

I usually start patients on L-tyrosine at 500 mg thirty minutes before breakfast and thirty minutes before lunch. I gradually increase the dose and find that 1,000–1,500 mg of L-tyrosine twice a day, thirty minutes before breakfast and lunch, is usually effective for many individuals with depression. However, I prefer N-acetyl tyrosine since it is better absorbed. One generally needs 500–1,000 mg two times a day.

Be sure and take 10 mg of vitamin B_6 after taking L-tyrosine. Also, some people taking L-tyrosine benefit from taking an additional 100–500 mcg a day of sublingual B_{12} and 1 mg of folic acid or 1 mg of MTHF or more a day.

DL-phenylalanine

DL-phenylalanine is another amino acid that is converted to tyrosine and leads to the production of neurotransmitters. Both tyrosine and phenylalanine have mood-elevating properties and may be beneficial along with 5-HTP. The dose of DL-phenylalanine usually is one to two 500-mg capsules in the morning on an empty stomach and one to two 500-mg capsules in the early afternoon on an empty stomach.

Mucuna. Traditionally used to treat depression or Parkinson's disease, this supplement contains up to 60 percent of levodopa. It has been shown to increase dopamine levels. Low dopamine is frequently associated with depression and apathy. Mucuna has been shown to raise dopamine levels and help with depression.[7] Mucuna pruriens is also known as velvet bean and has been used for centuries for improving mood and emotional well-being. I recommend Mucuna containing 60 percent L-Dopa in a 100-mg capsule. I recommend starting with one capsule in the morning thirty minutes before a meal. I do not recommend taking more than two capsules a day.

St. John's wort. This herb has been used for centuries to treat both depression and anxiety, with its medicinal uses first recorded in ancient Greece. An analysis of thirty-seven clinical trials concluded that St. John's wort may only provide minimal beneficial effects on *major* depression; however, the clinical trials did show greater benefits of St. John's wort for those with *minor* depression. The National Center for Complementary and Integrative Health (NCCIH) and the National Institutes of Health (NIH) say that St. John's wort was "no more effective than placebo in treating major depression of moderate severity."[8]

Therefore, I usually do not recommend St. John's wort for major depression. However, for mild depression or dysthymia, I usually recommend 300 mg of St. John's wort two or three times a day. If this is not effective after about three to four weeks, I usually have my patients double it to 600 mg two or three times a day. If patients do not see any benefits after two months, it probably will not help their depression. I must caution you not to take St. John's wort with any other antidepressants. HyperiMed is an excellent form of St. John's wort and can be found in many health food stores.

Supplements for anxiety

Now I would like to discuss a natural supplement protocol I recommend specifically for arming yourself against anxiety.

L-theanine

L-theanine is a unique amino acid that produces a relaxation effect on the brain similar to a mild tranquilizer. L-theanine is found in black tea, but higher concentrations are generally found in green tea—and the higher the quality of green tea, the higher the concentration of L-theanine.

A double-blind, placebo-controlled study of L-theanine in 2004 compared theanine with Xanax. Sixteen volunteers took either 1 mg of Xanax or 200 mg of theanine or placebo. Theanine, not the Xanax or placebo, induced relaxing effects that were evident at the initial measurement of whether a person felt tranquil versus troubled. Realize that 1 mg of Xanax is a significant dose, and most people use just 0.25 mg to 0.5 mg of Xanax.[9] So how does it work? Individuals experiencing anxiety, panic attacks, and insomnia usually have low levels of gamma-aminobutyric acid (GABA), an amino acid I will discuss next. Theanine actually helps produce a calming effect by boosting these GABA levels while it helps improve the mood by increasing levels of serotonin and dopamine.

In patients with anxiety, generalized anxiety disorder, and other anxiety disorders, I generally recommend about 100–200 mg of L-theanine one to three times a day.

L-theanine crosses the blood-brain barrier quite easily and does not cause drowsiness. However, because it does help people relax, I also recommend taking L-theanine at bedtime and find that it is effective in treating people with insomnia.

Gamma-aminobutyric acid (GABA)

GABA is an amino acid that also actually functions as a neurotransmitter in the brain. GABA and L-theanine are two of my favorite supplements for helping to relieve anxiety, and they usually work very well together.

Psychiatrists use benzodiazepines, such as Xanax, Ativan, and Valium, to control anxiety symptoms since these medications cross the blood-brain barrier and bind to GABA receptors in the brain, helping to alleviate anxiety. However, supplements of GABA and L-theanine have a brain-calming effect very similar to benzodiazepines without the addictive properties.

GABA generally works best when taken on an empty stomach about twenty or thirty minutes before a meal and taken only with water. I usually recommend 500–1,000 mg of GABA one to three times a day; many times I will combine it with L-theanine and 5 mg of vitamin B_6. However, individuals with severe anxiety may need even higher doses of GABA. GABA also seems to work best with vitamin B_6, and that is why it is so important to take a daily comprehensive multivitamin containing at least 2–10 mg of vitamin B_6.

Adaptogens

An adaptogen is a substance that will help the body adapt to stress by balancing the adrenal gland's response to stress. The end result is that cortisol levels will be neither too high nor too low but will be balanced. One I recommend is *Rhodiola rosea*, an herb native to the mountainous regions of Asia, parts of Europe, and the Arctic. I recommend a product that uses a standardization of 2–3 percent rosavin, the active ingredient of *Rhodiola* used in clinical studies. The common dose is 200–600 mg three times a day.

Others that can help you deal with stress and anxiety are ginseng, Korean ginseng (take 200 mg one to three times a day, three weeks on and two weeks off), Siberian ginseng, ashwagandha (3–6 gm a day), and magnolia bark.

For more recommendations for supplements to take for anxiety, see my book *The New Bible Cure for Depression and Anxiety.*

ARTHRITIS

The nutrients for overcoming arthritis include vitamins and supplements. Of course, these nutrients often are found in foods; they also may be taken as supplements. God has created living foods that prevent arthritis. But often our diets are inflammatory and are actually fueling the disease. Please refer to my books *The Bible Cure for Arthritis* and *Let Food Be Your Medicine* for the best diet for conquering arthritis.

Earlier I recommended taking a good multivitamin, but I want to emphasize the importance of this for arthritis sufferers. A comprehensive multivitamin is necessary in order to have proper amounts of vitamins and minerals that are required for the manufacture and maintenance of cartilage. The vitamins should contain adequate levels of the minerals zinc, copper, and boron, and also adequate levels of pantothenic acid, vitamin B_6, and vitamin A.

Osteoarthritis

If your osteoarthritis has reached the stage of chronic inflammation characterized by symptoms of swelling, stiffness, warmth, and pain, then you should immediately begin a diet of anti-inflammatory supplements, including curcumin, Boswellia, proteolytic enzymes, and glutathione booster supplements. One may take one of these anti-inflammatory supplements or a combination.

Curcumin

Curcumin is the active ingredient in turmeric that has powerful anti-inflammatory properties. Several studies imply that curcumin may ease symptoms of osteoarthritis and rheumatoid arthritis.[10] I typically recommend 500–1,000 mg of curcumin two to three times a day.

Boswellia

Boswellia has been used in Ayurvedic medicine as a natural anti-inflammatory for centuries. One study involved thirty participants with osteoarthritis of the knee who were treated with Boswellia extract or a placebo. All the patients in the Boswellia group reported a significant reduction in pain. Boswellia extract is usually standardized according to the concentration of boswellic acid in the product. Many studies have used the standardized boswellic acid concentration of no more than 40 percent. The usual dose of Boswellia is 300–400 mg three times a day.[11]

Proteolytic enzymes (Vascuzyme or Wobenzym)

Proteolytic enzymes are combinations of different proteolytic or protein-destroying enzymes, which are proteases. They were first developed in the 1950s by Professor Wolf and Dr. Benitez. Wobenzym was the product they developed. The ingredients include the plant enzymes bromelain and papain and the animal enzymes pancreatin, trypsin, and chymotrypsin. Numerous human and animal studies with subjects having arthritis and rheumatoid arthritis have shown that enzyme therapy can manage the symptoms of pain and inflammation as well as most conventional medicines but with none of the adverse effects. I typically recommend Vascuzyme or Wobenzym in a dose of three to four tablets on an empty stomach two to three times a day.[12] If you have ulcer disease or inflammation of the stomach or duodenum, you should not take proteolytic enzymes. Avoid proteolytic enzymes if you are pregnant.

RiboCeine

This powerful supplement helps reduce inflammation by boosting your body's natural glutathione production. I usually recommend two capsules of Cellgevity two times a day. (See appendix A.)

Krill oil

Krill oil contains fatty acids that help reduce or even neutralize the pro-inflammatory factors of arthritis. Krill oil comes from small crustaceans found in the icy waters of the Arctic and Antarctic Oceans. Krill oil is a richer source of DHA and EPA and is more easily absorbed compared to fish oil, so one needs fewer capsules. Krill oil is unlike fish oil because it also contains the powerful antioxidant astaxanthin that provides the red color and phospholipids that make the omega-3s more bioavailable, more stable, and with fewer lipid peroxides. In a study of krill oil combined with hyaluronic acid and astaxanthin, patients with arthritis reported pain reduction of 55 percent in less than three months, and 63 percent of those were completely pain-free. Krill oil is superior to fish oil at protecting joint cartilage from inflammation and actually accumulates in the joints. The dose of krill oil used in many of the arthritis studies was 300 mg, which I believe is a good starting dose.[13]

Type 2 collagen

Type 2 collagen is one of the key proteins in collagen. Taking type 2 collagen may improve symptoms of osteoarthritis by stimulating your body's own production of joint collagen. New research has found that osteoarthritis is due to an abnormal immune response to collagen proteins in the joint cartilage. However, oral type 2 collagen helps to desensitize the immune system to the collagen fibers, turning down or turning off the inflammatory response.[14] The dose is usually 40 mg of undenatured type 2 collagen on an empty stomach once a day.

- *Glucosamine and chondroitin sulfate*

Scientific research suggests the use of glucosamine sulfate in the treatment of osteoarthritis of the knee. Glucosamine is usually taken with chondroitin sulfate, which comes from cartilage.[15] The GAIT trial was the Glucosamine/chondroitin Arthritis Intervention Trial and tested the effects of glucosamine hydrochloride and chondroitin sulfate for the treatment of osteoarthritis of the knee. For a subset of patients with moderate to severe pain glucosamine/chondroitin gave statistically significant pain relief compared to a placebo.[16] I believe that they would have had better results had they used glucosamine sulfate instead of glucosamine hydrochloride. I typically recommend one tablet of a glucosamine chondroitin supplement containing 500 mg of glucosamine sulfate and 400 mg of chondroitin sulfate three times a day.

Hyaluronic acid (HA)

Hyaluronic acid is commonly taken for joint pain and arthritis because it can cushion joints and serve as a lubricant. Hyaluronic acid is a natural substance that is found in the synovial fluid of joints and functions as a lubricant and a shock absorber for joints. A study using an oral preparation of HA on obese knee osteoarthritis patients showed statistically significant improvements in pain and function.[17] I usually recommend low molecular weight HA in a dose of 200–400 mg a day in divided doses.

Fighting rheumatoid arthritis

Nutritional supplements for rheumatoid arthritis include a comprehensive multivitamin, which contain adequate amounts of B vitamins, minerals, and antioxidants such as vitamins C and E. Along with a multivitamin, consider taking the following supplements.

Proteolytic enzymes (Vascuzyme or Wobenzym)

Proteolytic enzymes are combinations of different proteolytic or protein-destroying enzymes, which are proteases. They were first developed in the 1950s by Professor Wolf and Dr. Benitez. Wobenzym was the product they developed. The ingredients include the plant enzymes bromelain and papain and the animal enzymes pancreatin, trypsin, and chymotrypsin. Numerous human and animal studies with subjects having arthritis and rheumatoid arthritis have shown that enzyme therapy can manage the symptoms of pain and inflammation as well as most conventional medicines but with none of the adverse effects.[18]

These enzymes usually have to be taken in a dose of four to five tablets, three times a day, between meals. However, you should be under the care of a nutritional doctor in order to manage this appropriately. If you have ulcer disease or inflammation of the stomach or duodenum, you should not take proteolytic enzymes. Avoid proteolytic enzymes if you are pregnant.

- *Curcumin*

This supplement comes from the yellow pigment of turmeric and has very strong anti-inflammatory properties. Several studies imply that curcumin may ease symptoms of osteoarthritis and rheumatoid arthritis.[19] The normal dose of curcumin is one to two capsules of 400–500 mg three times a day.

Type 2 Collagen

Type 2 collagen is a low molecular-weight hydrolyzed protein and is another very important nutrient for rebuilding cartilage. Collagen is the other main building block of cartilage, which is needed for the framework of the cartilage. Type 2 collagen has a unique structure that interfers with the inflammatory response and assists in reeducating the immune system. In a double blind placebo study of 60 patients with rheumatoid arthritis the number of swollen and tender joints decreased significantly in the type 2 collagen group and not in the placebo group, and 14 percent had a complete remission of their rheumatoid arthritis. Undenatured type 2 chicken collagen was used in the study.[20] The dose is usually 40 mg of undenatured type 2 collagen once a day on an empty stomach.

Boswellia

Boswellia limits inflammation by inhibiting the pro-inflammatory substance 5-LOX. Taking a supplement of Boswellia, especially with curcumin, can usually alleviate the symptoms of arthritis. Boswellia has been used in Ayurvedic medicine as a natural anti-inflammatory for centuries. One study involved thirty participants with osteoarthritis of the knee who were treated with Boswellia extract or a placebo. All the patients in the Boswellia group reported a significant reduction in pain. Boswellia extract is usually standardized according to the concentration of boswellic acid in the product. Many studies have used the standardized boswellic acid concentration of no more than 40 percent. The usual dose of Boswellia is 300–400 mg three times a day.[21]

RiboCeine

This powerful supplement helps reduce inflammation by boosting your body's natural glutathione production. I usually recommend two capsules of Cellgevity two times a day.

Hyaluronic acid (HA)

Hyaluronic acid is commonly taken for joint pain and arthritis because it can cushion joints and serve as a lubricant. Hyaluronic acid is a natural substance that is found in the synovial fluid of joints and functions as a lubricant and a shock absorber for joints. A study using an oral preparation of HA on obese knee osteoarthritis patients showed statistically significant improvements in pain and function.[22] I usually recommend low molecular weight HA in a dose of 200–400mg a day in divided doses.

Krill oil

Krill oil contains fatty acids that help reduce or even neutralize the pro-inflammatory factors of arthritis. Krill oil comes from small crustaceans found in the icy waters of the Arctic and Antarctic Oceans. Krill oil is a richer source of DHA and EPA and is more easily absorbed compared to fish oil, so one needs fewer capsules. Krill oil is unlike fish oil because it also contains the powerful antioxidant astaxanthin that provides the red color and phospholipids that make the omega-3s more bioavailable, more stable, and with fewer lipid peroxides. In a study of krill oil combined with hyaluronic acid and astaxanthin, patients with arthritis reported pain reduction of 55 percent in less than three months, and 63 percent of those were completely pain-free. Krill oil is superior to fish oil at protecting joint cartilage from inflammation and actually accumulates in the joints. The dose of krill oil used in many of the arthritis studies was 300 mg, which I believe is a good starting dose.[23]

The typical treatments for rheumatoid arthritis are nonsteroidal, anti-inflammatory medications. These include naproxen and ibuprofen. However, this class of drugs can further damage your intestinal tract, leading to increased intestinal permeability or leaky gut (intestines). This leads to worsening of food allergies since our bodies absorb whole-food proteins.

In rheumatoid arthritis the contrast to osteoarthritis is that you need to address the issues of poor digestion, increased intestinal permeability, food allergies, excessive inflammation, and adrenal fatigue. Refer to sections in this book on these subjects. This needs to be done by a nutritional doctor. You also need an antigen leukocyte cellular antibody test (ALCAT) to identify food sensitivities.

For both osteoarthritis and rheumatoid arthritis, one needs to alkalize his tissues by following an alkaline diet, drinking alkaline water, and taking supplements such as Vaxa's Buffer pH. The goal is to maintain a urine pH of 7.0–7.5.

ASTHMA

Natural supplements coupled with a proper diet not only will curtail asthma symptoms but also will make you feel better. Many natural supplements can be taken to help control the symptoms of asthma. I recommend you read

Reversing Inflammation and *Let Food Be Your Medicine* and follow the anti-inflammatory Mediterranean diet.

Antioxidants

Inflammation in the lungs leads to an influx of inflammatory cells, which, in turn, creates excessive amounts of free radicals, which I previously mentioned are highly reactive, highly charged particles that cause extensive cell damage in the body. Antioxidants are able to quench the free radicals and prevent significant tissue damage from taking place. Any asthma patient should have a rich supply of antioxidants in his body to counteract the work of the free radicals.

The most important antioxidant for the lungs is glutathione. When the lungs are under excessive oxidative stress, such as during an asthma attack, the glutathione levels decrease dramatically. However, RiboCeine can boost glutathione levels in the lungs when it is deficient. See appendix A.

A final important antioxidant is proanthocyanidin, otherwise known as grape seed, or pine bark extract. It is one of the most powerful antioxidants, fifty times more powerful than vitamin E and twenty times more powerful than vitamin C. Many European physicians have successfully used grape seed extract in treating hay fever and asthma because it helps prevent the release of histamine. I recommend 100–200 mg two to three times a day, taken on an empty stomach. You can find this at most health food stores.

Magnesium

Decades ago scientists discovered that magnesium sulfate worked as a natural bronchodilator. Although we now know that the primary cause of asthma is inflammation, not bronchial constriction, magnesium does help relax smooth muscles and dilate the bronchial tubes. Magnesium also functions as an anti-inflammatory agent to help stabilize mast cells.

An excellent blood test to determine if you are low in magnesium is the red blood cell (RBC) magnesium level. Most physicians check the regular serum magnesium test, which could show up as normal even if there is a problem. The RBC magnesium level is much more accurate, and many asthmatics will have a low RBC magnesium level.

I recommend a dosage of 200 mg of chelated magnesium two or three times a day.

Quercetin

Quercetin is a powerful bioflavonoid that acts as a strong antihistamine and anti-inflammatory supplement. It is also a powerful antioxidant that, like selenium, inhibits the release of leukotrienes. Quercetin is present in onions, garlic, and apples. I recommend a dose of 500 mg three times a day, to be gradually increased to a dose of 1,000 mg three to four times a day if needed.

Omega-3 fatty acids

Omega-3 fatty acids are better known as the fish oils. Foods rich in omega-3 acids can decrease levels of inflammatory-promoting compounds dramatically. Fish oil is incorporated into the fatty membrane that surrounds the cell and then works as a natural anti-inflammatory agent. I recommend at least 700–1,000 mg of omega-3 fatty acids three to four times per day. Be sure that any fish oil tablets that you take are not rancid. Many fish oil supplements sold at health food stores contain rancid oil. See appendix A. Caution: high dose fish oil may thin the blood and is contraindicated with blood thinners.

Moducare

Moducare contains plant sterols and sterolins that are usually missing in the standard American diet. It has immunomodulatory properties, which help reduce inflammation. Asthma patients should take one capsule of Moducare three times a day, thirty minutes to one hour before meals. It is available at many health food stores. Moducare also has a new chewable tablet for children.

AUTOIMMUNE DISORDERS

Supplements are a vital tool for providing your body with key nutrients that your body is lacking, which may be the reason why your body is not healing. Let's examine supplementation of vital nutrients that may provide some keys to your healing from autoimmune disease. I recommend you read the books *The Bible Cure for Autoimmune Diseases* and *Let Food Be Your Medicine* and follow the diet recommendations.

A comprehensive multivitamin

A comprehensive multivitamin is vitally important to provide the basic vitamins and minerals you need for optimum health. Unfortunately today's fast-food diet leaves our bodies starving for many essential vitamins and nutrients. And even the fresh fruits and vegetables we eat often are grown in nutrient-depleted soil.

Vitamins and minerals are essential components of your body that it cannot make for itself. It depends upon nutrition for them, but often you cannot get adequate amounts from the food you eat.

Some individuals with autoimmune disease may be sensitive to multivitamins and may be unable to take them until they have been desensitized, or they can take low doses every three to four days. If you get sick or nauseated when you take a multivitamin, consult a practitioner who can help.

Antioxidants

Those with autoimmune disease generally have far more inflammation and much more free-radical activity in their bodies. Therefore, taking certain antioxidant supplements every day is vitally important. Glutathione-boosting supplements are the most important for autoimmune disease. RiboCeine is the best glutathione-boosting supplement and is found in MaxOne and Cellgevity. See appendix A or one can take N-acetyl cysteine 500 mg–1,000 mg twice a day.

Sterols and sterolins

Moducare contains sterols and sterolins. These substances are plant fats. Recent research into Moducare has demonstrated that it has potent anti-inflammatory properties.[24]

Sterols and sterolins selectively activate and inhibit the immune system, which provides more effective control to a dysfunctional autoimmune response. Because the average American's diet is generally low in fruits and vegetables, many people lack these sterols and sterolins. Moducare supplies them.

To help modulate the immune response and decrease inflammation, I place many patients with autoimmune disease on Moducare. It is available at most health food stores.

Warning: Those with MS should not take Moducare since this may aggravate their condition.

Krill oil

Krill oil is high in omega-3 fatty acids, and supplementing with it for four weeks may raise eicosapentaenoic acid (EPA) and docosahexaenoic acid (DHA) levels. These fatty acids are useful in treating autoimmune disorders.[25] Krill is unlike omega-3s from fish oil because it also contains the powerful antioxident astaxanthin that provides the red color to krill. It also contains phospholipids that makes them more bioavailable, more stable, and with much fewer lipid peroxide, which are free radicals. I usually recommend krill 300 mg one to three tablets twice a day.

Curcumin

This supplement comes from the yellow pigment of turmeric and has very strong anti-inflammatory properties. The normal dose of curcumin is 40–1,000 mg two or three times a day.

Boswellia

This is an herb that may decrease inflammation and reduce autoimmune reactions.

Proteolytic enzymes

Autoimmune diseases often respond to systemic proteolytic enzymes. Immune complexes usually are involved in these diseases. These are substances formed when the body attacks what it believes is an outside invader, but in reality it is attacking itself. These substances, or complexes, attach to tissues in the body, eventually resulting in inflammation and possibly destruction of tissues. Proteolytic enzymes destroy immune complexes. It's important to take proteolytic enzymes between meals on an empty stomach.

I typically recommend Vascuzyme or Wobenzym three to four tablets two or three times a day on an empty stomach. (See my book *The Bible Cure for Autoimmune Diseases* for more information.)

Low-dose naltrexone

Low-dose naltrexone is usually very beneficial for patients with autoimmune disorders. It has been used in higher doses (50 mg) for decades to treat patients addicted to heroin, other opiates, and alcohol. When one takes low-dose naltrexone at bedtime, it helps prevent overactivity of the immune system, which is the root cause of autoimmune disease. The usual dose is 1.5–4.5 mg at bedtime. This is prescribed by a medical doctor.

BACK PAIN

Over the years I have treated thousands of patients with back pain. In medical school and during residency I was taught to prescribe anti-inflammatories, muscle relaxants, and pain medications. Using this regimen, most people overcame their back pain. Nevertheless, studies have shown that most back pain will go away in a few weeks, even without medication.[26] A much smaller group of people will go on to develop chronic back pain, which is sometimes severe enough to keep them from leading a normal, active, and vital lifestyle.

For back pain it is important to alkalize tissues by following an alkaline diet and drinking alkaline water.

One of the key restorative steps for those suffering from back pain is to get all the necessary vitamins, minerals, and other vital materials needed to adequately heal and repair any damage in your back's muscles, tissues, and bones.

There are special nutrients and supplements that can decrease inflammation, repair cartilage, help your muscles relax, and provide vital nutrients that may be missing.

Water

The most important nutrient for back pain is an adequate intake of water. Your back contains disks that are made up of a fibrous material called the *annulus fibrosis*. Inside is a jelly-like substance called the *nucleus pulposus*. This gel is made up mostly of water. As we age, the back's disks become dehydrated, which makes it increasingly easier to experience a herniated disk. Drink either two quarts of alkaline or spring water per day, or divide your body weight in pounds by two and drink that many ounces of water. Ideally your urine pH should be 7.0–7.5, which is indicative of how acidic your tissues are. If your urine pH is consistently higher than 8.0, choose more spring water or less alkaline water.

Glucosamine and chondroitin sulfate

An important supplement for back pain is glucosamine and chondroitin sulfate, taken separately or combined into one tablet.

Glucosamine sulfate is an amino sugar, which is actually made from the sugar glucose and the amino acid glutamine. It helps prevent osteoarthritis and can build joint cartilage.

Chondroitin sulfate is a mucopolysaccharide that helps form cartilage tissue, as well as attracting and holding water in the cartilage tissue in order to maintain healthy cartilage. A combination tablet of glucosamine and chondroitin typically contains 500 mg of glucosamine and 400 mg of chondroitin and should be taken three times a day.

Proteolytic enzymes

This is a powerful, natural substance that contains plant and animal enzymes. Bromelain is found in pineapples and has anti-inflammatory effects. Proteolytic enzymes such as Wobenzym and Vascuzyme help reduce pain, inflammation, and swelling.[27] Both bromelain and proteolytic enzymes are best taken between meals, approximately thirty minutes to one hour before meals or two hours after meals.

I usually recommend three to four Wobenzym or Vascuzyme tablets two or three times a day on an empty stomach. However, if you have an ulcer or gastritis or are taking other prescription anti-inflammatory medications, I do not recommend that you take these supplements.

NOTE: Avoid proteolytic enzymes and bromelain if you are pregnant.

Multivitamins

A comprehensive multivitamin/mineral is important to be sure that you are getting enough of the necessary basic vitamins, minerals, and antioxidants to maintain health.

Other supplements for back pain

Some other supplements, many of which treat arthritis, also may be useful in treating back pain:

- *Curcumin*

This substance found in turmeric has an anti-inflammatory agent and may help with pain. I usually recommend curcumin 500–1,000 mg one capsule two to three times a day.

Boswellia

This limits inflammation by inhibiting the pro-inflammatory substance 5-LOX. Taking a supplement of Boswellia can alleviate symptoms. The usual dose of Boswellia is 300–400mg two to three times a day.

RiboCeine

This powerful nutrient helps reduce inflammation by boosting your body's natural glutathione production. See appendix A for Cellgevity. You may take one capsule twice a day or N-acetyl cysteine 500–1000 mg twice a day.

Krill oil

This contains fatty acids that help reduce or even neutralize the pro-inflammatory factors of arthritis and joint pain. I usually start patients on krill oil 300 mg or more a day and may increase the dose if needed.

Type 2 collagen

This can help reduce joint pain. More research is needed, but type 2 collagen is said to help pain and inflammation because it causes the body to make substances that counteract inflammation.[28] The dose is usually 40 mg a day on an empty stomach.

Hyaluronic acid

This is commonly taken for joint pain and arthritis because it can cushion joints and serve as a lubricant.

CANCER

One of the tools in fighting cancer is supplements, which we should add to our regimen to make sure we are getting what we need every day. It can be hard to plan your daily meals to include every food you should eat to get the maximum anticancer benefits, but by adding a daily supplement regimen of phytonutrients, supplements that boost the immune system, and anticancer nutrients, you can have a great deal of protection from their benefits alone. These are often called *phytonutrients*. They have existed in our foods since God first created the earth, and science is just beginning to discover their incredible potential.

Exciting, isn't it? You probably want to know more about the phytonutrients and supplements you need to live healthily, fight disease, and avoid cancer, and how to get them into your daily diet. Well, here's the info you need! (These supplements are recommended for any type of cancer and are presented in no special order.)

While I will review various beneficial vitamins, minerals, and nutrients, it is important to remember that fighting cancer starts with being healthy and maintaining a healthy, strong immune system. Research shows that from a young age, your body handles fifty to one hundred thousand mutated—i.e., potentially cancerous—cells almost every day of your life, but it is only as your body and its tissues and organs become stressed with age, lack of sleep, being overweight, not getting enough exercise, poor diet, smoking, too much stress from work or life, an excessive toxic burden, and compromised liver function that cancer can get a foothold in your body. I strongly recommend *The Seven Pillars of Health* to learn more about these issues. Staying at a healthy weight, getting adequate rest, coping with stress, exercising regularly, eating a healthy diet, and getting the proper recommended daily allowances of the correct nutrients is the best plan for keeping cancer out of your life or conquering it.

Comprehensive multivitamin (with minerals)

Every good health-promoting supplement routine should start with a comprehensive multivitamin and mineral.

So find a high-quality, comprehensive daily multivitamin with minerals to use as the basis of your supplement routine. Many multivitamins are divided by gender or according to health concerns, so make sure to add to those the individual supplements that are needed for your particular concerns or health issues.

Selenium

Selenium and sulfur are part of glutathione peroxidase, the body's most important antioxidant and detoxifying agent. Animal studies have shown that selenium helps inhibit the formation of tumors and also may slow their growth.

Selenium is a very important mineral for our bodies, yet most Americans only get between 60 mcg and 100 mcg of it a day instead of the recommended 200 mcg.[29] This mineral helps prevent damaged DNA molecules from replicating and repeating the mistakes that become cell mutations. More than one hundred studies have been done with animals and have shown selenium to be a powerful preventative of tumor formations. In human trials it also has been shown as a strong preventative as well as slowing existing cancers, particularly prostate cancer. In one study it cut the incidence of lung cancer by nearly 50 percent.[30] While research continues on this valuable mineral, it is not too early to make sure you are getting the daily recommended amount of it in your multivitamin. I recommend 200 mcg a day of selenium.

Vitamin D_3

Is it possible that sunlight could be a preventative to cancer? Recent research seems to indicate that higher levels of vitamin D, which the skin will manufacture in our bodies when exposed to sunlight, may reduce the risk of breast, prostate, and other cancers by as much as 66 percent. Vitamin D helps repair DNA mutations.

In the Nurses Health Study, done with 1,760 nurses, coauthor Cedric Garland said:

> The data is very clear, showing that individuals in the group with the lowest blood levels had the highest rates of breast cancer, and the breast cancer rates dropped as the blood levels of 25-hydroxyvitamin D increased.... The serum level associated with a 50 percent reduction in risk could be maintained by taking 2,000 international units of vitamin D_3 daily, plus, when the weather permits, spending 10 to 15 minutes a day in the sun.[31]

JoEllen Welsh, a researcher at the State University of New York at Albany, has been conducting research on vitamin D for twenty-five years. She found that when mice injected with breast cancer cells were treated with vitamin D, after several weeks the tumors shrank by 50 percent, and some even disappeared.[32]

Of a study published in the *American Journal of Preventive Medicine* in 2007, study coauthor Edward Gorham said:

> Through this meta-analysis we found that raising the serum level of 25-hydroxyvitamin D to 34 ng/ml would reduce the incidence of colorectal cancer by half.... We project a two-thirds reduction in incidence with serum levels of 46 ng/ml, which corresponds to a daily intake of 2,000 IU of vitamin D_3. This would be best achieved with a combination of diet, supplements and 10 to 15 minutes per day in the sun.[33]

I advocate following their advice and adding 2,000–5,000 IU of vitamin D_3 to your daily supplements. I also check 25OHD3 serum levels and adjust the patient's dose of vitamin D_3 until I reach a level of 50–80 ng/ml. The patient with low levels of vitamin D_3 may need to take 5,000 units of vitamin D_3 a day for three to four months and then have their vitamin D_3 level rechecked. Most patients eventually can be maintained on a dose of 2,000–4,000 IU a day.

Omega-3 fatty acids (EPA and DHA)

A higher intake of omega-3 fatty acids, obtained through eating cold-water fish, such as salmon and sardines, or more conveniently through taking pharmaceutical-grade fish oil capsules, has been linked with lower inflammation and lower cancer risk, as well as a multitude of other health benefits. There is good evidence that these fatty acids repair cells and DNA, keeping mutations from being made in cellular reproduction. They work to "switch off" production of molecules necessary to the cancer cycle and "switch on" genes that signal for apoptosis (cell death) in cells before they can become full-blown tumors.

Due to these positive effects, I encourage taking a daily fish oil supplement that is not rancid. A good dosage for most people to include with their normal supplements would be 300–1,000 mg three times a day. Caution: fish oil thins the blood and should not be taken with other blood thinners unless cleared by one's medical doctor. (See appendix A.)

Curcumin

Curcumin, the valuable compound found in the spice turmeric, may help prevent or fight prostate, pancreatic, breast, and colon cancers. It probably does this because curcumin inhibits the cyclooxygenase-2 (COX-2) enzyme that promotes inflammation. (Aspirin also inhibits the COX-2 enzyme and helps prevent colon cancer.) Research has shown that curcumin can remove ten different cancer-causing factors. Curcumin can do the following:

- Block nuclear factor-kappaB, a molecule causing inflammation
- Disrupt the body's production of advanced glycation end products, which cause inflammation
- Enhance the control of replication of cells
- Encourage cell death in cancer cells that are quickly reproducing
- Increase the vulnerability of tumors
- Increase the death of cancer cells by regulating pathways of tumor suppressors
- Limit the invasiveness of tumors
- Block "pathways to penetration of tissue"
- Reduce the blood supply of tumors
- Limit the ability of cancer to spread[34]

Curcumin also can be taken in supplement form. Remember that it is an antioxidant several times more powerful than vitamin E. Piperine, a compound found in pepper, increases its absorption. Because of this and the incredible health benefits of curcumin for multiple diseases, I suggest you have 500–1,000 mg of curcumin one to three times a day in a supplement that also includes piperine to increase its absorption.

Melatonin

Melatonin has long been touted as a natural sleep aid, but did you know it also has significant anticancer benefits? Melatonin has been shown to improve immune system function, help individuals cope with stress, and diminish certain aspects of aging, as well as help fight fibrocystic breast diseases and breast and colon cancers. Low melatonin levels are associated with cancer. Melatonin helps to inhibit tumor growth in humans and helps to prevent the spread of cancer by anti-angiogenesis properties. It also demonstrates protection against the toxic side effects of chemotherapy and radiation therapy and improves healing after cancer surgery.[35] Those who already sleep well may not need a melatonin supplement to help their natural production of it. For more information on melatonin, please refer to *The New Bible Cure for Sleep Disorders*. I usually recommend 1–20 mg of melatonin dissolved in the mouth at bedtime or if you awaken during the night. Start low and go slow. Melatonin can cause vivid dreams, grogginess the next day, and brain fog in some patients.

Diindolylmethane (DIM) and Indole-3-Carbinol (I3C)

Indole-3-carbinol (I3C), one of the powerful compounds found in cruciferous vegetables that the body turns into valuable diindolylmethane (DIM), also can be taken in supplement form. DIM is the most active cruciferous substance for promoting healthy estrogen metabolism. While this does not change the value of your grandmother's advice to "Eat your broccoli, cauliflower, and brussels sprouts!" it can still help you get some of their most effective benefits without struggling to chew them up and swallow them. These compounds seem especially beneficial for those at risk of the hormone-driven cancers of the breasts, ovaries, uterus, prostate, and cervix. Because they modulate estrogen, pregnant women should avoid these supplements, but for others concerned with hormone-driven cancers, you should take a daily supplement of cruciferous vegetable extracts. I usually recommend 100 mg of DIM two times a day and/or 120 mg of I3C twice a day. DIM is more stable than I3C, so it is preferable.

Calcium D-glucarate

Calcium D-glucarate is a natural detoxifier and supports the body's detox systems. It is extracted from fruits such as apples, oranges, and grapefruit and from cruciferous vegetables, such as broccoli and brussels sprouts.

In order to eliminate certain toxins and hormones from our bodies, glucuronic acid is attached to them in the liver and then excreted in the bile. D-glucarate inhibits beta-glucuronidase, which is a bacterial enzyme that promotes hormone-driven cancers, such as breast, prostate, and colon cancers. It also may reduce the risk of lung, liver, skin, and other types of cancers. I recommend a supplement including 200 mg of calcium D-glucarate a day with or without food.

Glutathione

As has previously been stated, glutathione is the most important antioxidant in the body. It also functions as a detoxifier of the body, neutralizing toxins and heavy metals as well as quenching free radicals. The reduced form of glutathione is the active form and is abbreviated as GSH. Glutathione is water soluble and concentrated mainly in the blood and cytoplasm portion of every cell in your body. The liver has the highest per-cell concentration of glutathione.

Also, vitamin D_3, according to scientific literature, decreases levels of glutathione and increases production of free radicals in every type of cancer cell. In other words, one way vitamin D_3 protects us against cancer is by robbing the cancer cell of glutathione, which usually protects the cancer cell from destruction.

I recommend glutathione-promoting supplements to everyone who wants to prevent cancer. Refer to appendix A.

The power of enzymes

Though his theories are still largely controversial, the story of dentist William Kelley is a testimony to the power of diet, nutrients, enzymes, and detoxification in the treatment and prevention of cancer. Dr. Kelley was diagnosed with inoperable pancreatic cancer in 1967 and was told he had only months to live. In response he began experimenting with the regimen of a natural foods diet, proper supplements, high-dose enzyme therapy, and a detox program that cleansed him of toxins. This cured him of the deadly cancer he faced. Not only that, but also he lived on until the age of seventy-nine, passing away in 2005, roughly thirty-eight years after his diagnosis. Kelley's method also worked for thousands of others over that time. His book *One Answer to Cancer* is still widely referenced today. His theories were based on the work of Dr. John Beard, who published *The Enzyme Theory of Cancer* in 1911.

Kelley believed that cancer was a pancreatic-enzyme deficiency caused by the body being overloaded with secondhand proteins (from the meats we eat), and thus the enzymes were not able to digest the foreign proteins known as cancer. There are twenty-two different types of enzymes produced in the body, most of them by the pancreas. This production is one of the things that wane as we grow older. Chronic enzyme deficiency weakens the immune system. It is possible to replace such enzymes through the foods we eat and by taking proteolytic and digestive enzyme supplements.

Cancer cells, like nearly all pathogens, are enclosed in fibrin, a protein-based coating that makes it difficult for the immune system to recognize. It is fifteen times thicker than the membranes of normal cells. When there are enough of these digestive enzymes floating around in our systems, they will eat through that thick cell membrane and expose cancer to the arresting power of the immune system; when enzymes are not there, cancers can go undetected and undeterred.

The late Dr. Nicholas Gonzalez studied Kelley's research and patients as a medical school student and is one of the main proponents of enzyme therapy today. His tests with it, however, have yet to live up to the results in Kelley's life and in the lives of some of his patients; thus what has come to be known as "the Kelley Protocol" is still largely under debate. There are still nutritionists, naturopaths, and other nutritional doctors who monitor patients on the Kelley Protocol in managing cancer. I do not recommend this program unless you are being followed by a doctor trained in the Kelley Protocol.

Regardless, I believe proteolytic enzyme therapy and the Kelley Protocol are still worth considering, especially what Kelley believed about the foods we eat and keeping our bodies detoxified. If you are facing cancer, it certainly would be worth looking further into the research and discussing enzyme therapy with a nutritional doctor. Smaller doses of digestive enzymes also may have health benefits for those looking at them as a preventative supplement to be taken with meals. I personally take three to four proteolytic enzymes each morning on an empty stomach.

It is also beneficial to eat healthy in the fight against cancer. Read *The New Bible Cure for Cancer*, and follow the dietary recommendations.

Candida/Yeast Infections

A number of natural herbs and supplements are powerfully effective against candida. Begin supplementing a healthy diet with sources of good bacteria. The lining of your gastrointestinal (GI) tract has been a war zone and will need to be repaired, and any parasitic infestations you may have also must be addressed. Let's look at some supplements that can help, and most of these supplements can be found in a health food store or online.

Garlic

One of the most important supplements for controlling yeast overgrowth is garlic. Allicin, the active ingredient in garlic, has powerful antifungal activity. Take 500 mg of garlic three times a day.

Goldenseal/Berberine

Goldenseal is included in the same family with Oregon grape and barberry. They are all in the berberine family. These potent natural substances contain extremely effective antifungal agents. These special agents actually activate macrophages, which are a type of white blood cell.

Berberines help clear out bacterial overgrowth in the small intestines, which commonly accompanies yeast overgrowth. Berberines also halt the bacterial and yeast enzymes that aggravate leaky gut. Many patients with chronic candidiasis have diarrhea. Berberines are also able to control diarrhea in many cases. Take 500 mg of goldenseal three times a day for at least a month.

Grapefruit seed extract

Grapefruit seed extract, otherwise known as citrus extract, is a great supplement for candida. It effectively kills both the candida and the parasite giardia, which may be associated with candida in some cases. However, it usually takes several months to eliminate the parasites. Take 100–200 mg of grapefruit seed extract three times a day.

Caprylic acid

Caprylic acid is a long-chain fatty acid found in coconuts. It's extremely toxic to yeast, yet safe for humans. To be effective it must be taken in a time-released capsule. Take 1,000 mg of a time-released preparation with each meal.

Oil of oregano

Oil of oregano is a very good antifungal agent. It's more than one hundred times more potent than caprylic acid. I recommend oregano oil tablets. Take two to three 50-mg tablets of oregano three times a day.

Tanalbit

Tanalbit is a plant extract that destroys yeast, including the spores, without harming good bacteria. It also contains natural tannins, which have intestinal antiseptic properties.

Take three capsules three times a day, with each meal.

Chlorophyll supplements (green food)

Chlorophyll supplements, otherwise known as green food supplements, detoxify the colon and pack a powerful punch against candida. They boost the immune system as well. Chlorophyll keeps yeast and bacteria from spreading, and it even encourages the growth of friendly bacteria and helps repair the intestinal tract.

High-chlorophyll foods include wheat grass, barley grass, alfalfa, chlorella, spirulina, and blue/green algae. All of these are obtained in Divine Health Fermented Green Supremefood. Fermentation predigests the grasses and vegetables and adds probiotics, improving digestion and absorption. These high-chlorophyll foods are very nutrient-dense and are excellent sources of essential amino acids, vitamins, minerals, essential fatty acids, and phytonutrients.

High-chlorophyll foods not only boost the immune system, but they also help improve both digestion and elimination and help repair the gastrointestinal (GI) tract, usually damaged from candida overgrowth.

Probiotics

Probiotics, or friendly bacteria, have many benefits, including producing fatty acids that make it difficult for candida to survive. Good bacteria coat the lining of the intestines, forming a protective barrier against invasions by yeast and other microorganisms. Here are some types of good bacteria.

Lactobacillus acidophilus

Lactobacillus acidophilus is powerful against the growth of candida. This good form of bacteria lives in your small intestines all the time.

You can be sure that your body has enough of these important bacteria by drinking lactose-free kefir or by eating lactose-, fruit-, and sugar-free yogurt. During a severe attack of candida overgrowth, you also can choose to supplement with good bacteria.

The DDS-1 strain of lactobacillus acidophilus is a super-efficient strain of acidophilus, which is superior in its ability to attach to the lining of the small intestines and help control yeast overgrowth. DDS-1 is a supplement that can be found in most health food stores. It is important to keep it refrigerated. Take one teaspoon one or two times a day on an empty stomach.

Fructooligosaccharides (FOS)

FOS is a special polysaccharide that is not digested by man yet feeds friendly bacteria and helps them to grow, while at the same time reducing bad bacteria.

Take 2,000 mg of FOS a day in order to nourish the good bacteria. You can find FOS at any health food store. It is commonly combined with the acidophilus and bifidus supplements.

You should take at least 20–50 billion colony-forming units of acidophilus and bifidus bacteria on a daily basis in order to recolonize the GI tract. This usually will enable your body to overcome yeast. I also recommend that patients take one tablespoon of chia seeds in 8 ounces of water twice a day to rid the GI tract of candida.

Some patients may need nystatin and/or Diflucan for moderate to severe cases of candida, which are prescribed by a medical doctor.

CHRONIC FATIGUE AND FIBROMYALGIA

Since most patients with fibromyalgia and chronic fatigue have significant adrenal fatigue, I always place them on supplements that support the adrenal glands.

Supplements for adrenal fatigue

There are many types of supplements to help support and restore the adrenal glands, and I explain them in the adrenal fatigue section. I will list here my favorite supplements for adrenal fatigue, especially for those suffering from fibromyalgia and chronic fatigue syndrome (CFS).

A multivitamin

Take a comprehensive multivitamin that contains adequate amounts of magnesium, niacin, and B_6, which are important cofactors in converting 5-hydroxytryptophan (5-HTP) to serotonin.

B-complex vitamins

Deficiency in any or all of the B vitamins is commonly associated with fatigue and sleep disturbances, eventually resulting in atrophy of the adrenal glands. Vitamin B_5 (pantothenic acid) is especially important because it plays a significant part in the production of adrenal hormones; it is sometimes called the antistress vitamin. I recommend taking a B-complex vitamin one to two times a day. But do not take B-complex 100, which contains 100 mg of most of the B vitamins. Dosages of vitamin B_6 of 100 mg or greater can cause neuropathy.

Minerals

Low magnesium levels are very common in individuals with adrenal fatigue. Increased stress as well as adrenal fatigue cause our bodies to have an increased need for magnesium. The dietary recommendation for magnesium is 300 mg. I commonly recommend 200 mg of magnesium two times a day.

Dehydroepiandrosterone (DHEA)

This is involved in many processes in the human body. It promotes the growth and repair of protein tissue, especially muscle, and it acts to regulate cortisol, negating many of the harmful effects of ongoing excessive cortisol. A depressed level of DHEA may serve as an early warning sign of adrenal exhaustion. I recommend either 7-keto DHEA or DHEA in a dose of approximately 50 mg a day for men or 25 mg a day for women. Some DHEA is converted to estrogen. However, 7-keto DHEA does not convert to estrogen.

Pregnenolone

Pregnenolone is made largely from cholesterol, which is used, in turn, to make DHEA. It is known as the "hormone balancer" since it has the ability to increase levels of steroid hormones that are deficient in the body and can decrease excessive levels of circulating hormones. Supplementation can be beneficial for many people who experience the symptoms of chronic fatigue and fibromyalgia. There is not a standard dosage of pregnenolone, but it is typically given at 30 mg on a daily basis.[36]

Adrenal glandular supplements

These contain protomorphogens or extracts of tissues from the adrenal glands of pigs or cattle. These can be taken orally to support human adrenal function. Each organ of the body has a unique mix of vitamins, minerals, and hormones. Glandular substances in pigs and cattle have an "adrenal mix" close to that of the human adrenal glands. Some doctors of natural medicine have used adrenal glandular supplements with their patients for decades and report very positive results. De-Stress Formula (DSF) is one such supplement, and I recommend one to two tabs two times per day, with breakfast and lunch, or Drenamin from Standard Process three tablets twice a day.

Progesterone (for women)

As women age, the ovaries gradually produce less and less progesterone, and eventually the production ceases around menopause. In even younger women suffering from severe adrenal fatigue, cortisol levels are typically low, as are progesterone levels. This is because the body robs progesterone from the ovaries to produce cortisol, which becomes depleted under long-term stress. Some women benefit from bioidentical progesterone supplementation using transdermal creams or an oral dose of progesterone at bedtime if the patient has insomnia. If women test low for female hormones, I recommend a bioidentical progesterone cream. This is a prescription and must be prescribed by a physician.

Adaptogens

Adaptogens are substances that will help the body adapt to stress by balancing cortisol levels. They help the body's mental and physical performance while providing resistance to stressful insults at the cellular level. Adaptogens include *Rhodiola*, Korean ginseng, Siberian ginseng, ashwagandha, and epimedium. More information can be found in my book *Stress Less*.

Supplements for energy

Over-the-counter energy supplements, such as caffeine and most energy drinks, usually stress the adrenal glands, but I have found a few key supplements that increase one's energy without stressing and draining adrenal function.

Glutathione-boosting supplements

Glutathione helps maintain your body's energy-producing mitochondria and enables the mitochondria to produce optimal amounts of adenosine triphosphate (ATP) by quenching free radicals. ATP is the energy currency in the body.

Glutathione is produced in your body and recycled by your body all the time—except chronic diseases, including chronic fatigue syndrome (CFS) and fibromyalgia, usually deplete the glutathione in our bodies. As a consequence, patients with CFS and fibromyalgia often have very low energy. If oxidative stress or toxins overwhelm your body, your glutathione levels drop and your body's protection against free radicals, infections, and illnesses becomes greatly compromised. It becomes harder for your body to get rid of the toxins as well. This creates a vicious cycle of chronic illness.

Studies have found that people with chronic fatigue syndrome are usually depleted in glutathione, and boosting their intracellular glutathione levels may help their symptoms improve.[37] I recommend glutathione-boosting supplements to every patient with chronic fatigue or fibromyalgia. N-acetyl cysteine 500 mg or MaxOne are good supplements. Take one capsule of either two times per day.

D-ribose

D-ribose is a simple 5-carbon sugar that helps the body produce new ATP. Supplementing with D-ribose in one study increased the total amount of ATP produced by up to four.[38] I recommend usually one scoop two or three times a day in water or green tea.

Acetyl L-carnitine and alpha lipoic acid

Acetyl L-carnitine boosts the conversion of fats into energy in the mitochondria. Alpha lipoic acid also is involved in mitochondrial ATP production and can recycle other antioxidants. Together they work synergistically. I recommend 500–1,000 mg one or two times a day of acetyl L-carnitine and 300 mg of alpha lipoic acid twice a day.

Nicotinamide adenine dinucleotide hydrate (NADH)

NADH may increase energy significantly in some patients. NADH plays a role in the biochemical processes that generate energy. I recommend 5–10 mg two times a day. This supplement, however, is quite expensive and doesn't help everyone.

Coenzyme Q_{10} (CoQ_{10})

CoQ_{10} helps increase ATP (energy) and is especially effective when combined with pyrroloquinoline quinone (PQQ). Ubiquinol is the biologically superior form of CoQ_{10}. I recommend 100–200 mg of CoQ_{10} two times a day.

Pyrroloquinoline quinone (PQQ)

PQQ is an antioxidant compound that is emerging as the micronutrient that may reverse cellular aging. It plays an essential role in defending cells against mitochondrial decay. PQQ's chemical structure enables it to withstand exposure to oxidation up to five thousand times greater than vitamin C. It not only protects mitochondria from damage, but it also stimulates growth of new mitochondria. I recommend 20 mg once or twice per day. I personally take Max ATP, PQQ, and ubiquinol to boost my energy.

Methylcobalamin

Methylcobalamin, or the active form of vitamin B_{12} that is used by the central nervous system, helps boost energy. I usually recommend 100 mcg to 1 mg per day.

Myers IV

The Myers IV helps restore adrenal function. Nutrients in a Myers IV include magnesium chloride, calcium gluconate, methylcobalamin, pyridoxine hydrochloride, pantothenic acid, vitamin B_5, vitamin B_6, B-complex, and buffered vitamin C. I usually give this IV to my patients with chronic fatigue and fibromyalgia once a week.

Royal Jelly

If energy is not increasing, I recommend Royal Jelly. This supplement comes from bees, which use it to nurture the queen bee. Its composition is altered based on where it is produced, but it does contain water, proteins, vitamins, and more.[39] It is used for many disorders, including increasing energy. I recommend an eighth to a quarter of a teaspoon one or two times per day. Keep refrigerated.

If one has chronic fatigue or fibromyalgia that is not improved with these nutrients, I strongly recommend testing for mold toxins and lyme disease. Refer to Dr. Ritchie Shoemaker's book *Surviving Mold*.

COLDS, FLU, AND SINUS INFECTIONS

Your body needs to maintain a good, steady supply of basic vitamins and minerals to maintain its fighting edge. Today's modern diet does not always provide all the essentials. In fact, even if your diet is rich with fruits and vegetables, there's a good chance they were grown on depleted soil. Therefore, to maintain the strength and power of your immune system, take a good multivitamin/mineral supplement every day. Also, follow an anti-inflammatory diet, and if you have frequent colds and sinus infections, avoid sugar and dairy. Once your immune system has recovered and you are free of colds and sinus infections, then rotate dairy every four days. If infections return, then avoid dairy.

A comprehensive multivitamin/mineral

Certain vitamins and minerals are critically important for your immune system to function at peak efficiency, which is vital during cold and flu season. A comprehensive multivitamin is very important to provide the basic vitamins and minerals for your body that it cannot make for itself. You cannot get adequate amounts from the food you eat. Therefore, I recommend a comprehensive multivitamin/mineral supplement such as Divine Health's

Enhanced Multivitamin. It provides essential vitamins and minerals as well as most of the antioxidants your body requires on a daily basis.

Vitamin A

If your body lacks enough vitamin A, you will tend to be very prone to many types of infections, especially colds and flu. Vitamin A works to maintain the structural integrity of the mucous membranes. It's also vitally important in the production of T-cells.

A deficiency of vitamin A actually will cause your thymus gland to shrink, resulting in an impaired immune system. Many physicians are concerned about vitamin A overdosing since it's associated with liver damage, loss of hair, headaches, vomiting, and other symptoms. Yet vitamin A overdosing is extremely rare, but inadequate consumption of vitamin A is very common.

I recommend 5,000–10,000 IU of vitamin A every day, which is a safe dosage. However, if you are pregnant, limit your dosage to 5,000 IU of vitamin A per day.

Some people believe they don't need vitamin A because they take supplements of beta-carotene. They reason that since beta-carotene is a precursor to vitamin A, it's all they really need. However, vitamin A, beta-carotene, and other carotenoids all have independent roles to play in strengthening and protecting immunity. Therefore, all these nutrients should be taken regularly. Vitamin A is present in most multivitamins.

B-complex

B vitamins are also very important for optimal immune function. Vitamin B_5, or pantothenic acid, is important for maintaining a healthy thymus gland and for antibody production. Folic acid is important for optimal function of T-cells and B-cells, as is vitamin B_6. Vitamin B_{12} is needed by phagocytes to kill bacteria.

Vitamin C

Vitamin C is also extremely important for the immune system. Vitamin C is both an antiviral and antibacterial agent. Vitamin C strengthens connective tissue and also neutralizes toxic substances that are released from phagocytes.

In 1970 Dr. Linus Pauling released the book *Vitamin C and the Common Cold*.[40] He was one of the most prominent and respected scientists of the twentieth century and had been awarded two Nobel prizes. But he stirred up tremendous controversy in the medical community when he recommended that people take 1,000–2,000 mg of vitamin C daily for general well-being. To fight a cold, he recommended upping the dosage to 4,000–10,000 mg a day.

Dr. Pauling found that supplementing with 1,000 mg of vitamin C daily reduced the incidence of colds by 45 percent and reduced cold symptoms by 63 percent.[41] As a preventive dose, I recommend 1,000 mg of vitamin C taken daily, preferably 250 mg three to four times a day or 500 mg twice a day. If you have a cold or sinus infection, I recommend boosting your dosage to 2,000 mg of vitamin C, preferably in powdered form, every two to three hours. Maintain this dosage for several days, and then gradually taper off until you're back to 1,000 mg a day as a maintenance dose.

Taking over 3,000 mg of vitamin C at one time is likely to produce diarrhea and gas. If you experience such symptoms, decrease your dose to only 500–1,000 mg. In rare instances high doses of vitamin C can cause kidney stones; therefore, it's critically important to drink at least two quarts of water a day.

Consult with your physician before starting a high-dose vitamin C therapy.

Vitamin D

Research has shown that vitamin D may be as effective as Vitamin C when fighting or preventing colds. Individuals with low vitamin D levels tend to have more colds than those with normal levels. Nineteen thousand individuals participated in this study by having their vitamin D levels tested and reporting colds and respiratory infections. Those with vitamin D levels lower than 10 ng/ml were 36 percent more likely to have recently had a cold than those with vitamin D levels higher than 30 ng/ml.[42] Most of my patients take 2,000–5,000 IU of vitamin D_3 a day. Have your vitamin D_3 level checked to make sure you are taking enough vitamin D_3.

Selenium

Minerals are also vitally important for good immune function. One of the most important minerals for building and maintaining superior immunity is selenium. Selenium deficiency causes a reduction in T-cell activity and antibody production.

It also can lower your resistance to developing viral and bacterial infections. Selenium supplements significantly enhance the body's production of white blood cells—especially T-cells and natural killer cells.

Take approximately 200 mcg of selenium a day. A comprehensive multivitamin usually contains selenium.

Zinc

Zinc is another very important mineral for the immune system. In fact, it's vital to the function of the thymus gland and is required for cell-mediated immunity. A deficiency in zinc will cause a decrease in T-cells, natural killer cells, and thymic hormone. In test tubes zinc has been found to prevent cold viruses from reproducing themselves.

A study on zinc throat lozenges found that the recovery times were shorter for subjects who, when they were developing cold symptoms, dissolved zinc lozenges in their mouths every two hours. The average recovery time for those who took the lozenges was 4.4 days, while that increased to 7.6 days for those who were given a placebo.[43]

Most American diets are low in zinc. Some experts believe our low zinc intake is the reason so many of us have immune problems. Nevertheless, all zinc is not equal. Zinc gluconate or zinc acetate is preferred to zinc picolinate or zinc citrate. Make sure that your zinc throat lozenges do not contain sugar or tartrate fillers, since zinc binds to these fillers and becomes less available.

If you use zinc throat lozenges, it's important that you begin within twenty-four hours of the first sign of symptoms for the maximum benefit. Zinc is present in a comprehensive multivitamin. I recommend at least 15 mg a day.

Natural remedies

Let's turn now and look at some natural remedies that can help you beat the symptoms of a cold, flu, or sinus infection.

Elderberry

Native Americans also used tea made from elderberry flowers to treat respiratory infections. Elderberry extract, which has a large amount of three flavonoids, has been shown to help treat viruses.

A study published in the *Journal of Alternative and Complementary Medicine* in 1995 examined the flu-fighting capabilities of Sambucol, which is an elderberry extract preparation. The study found that elderberry inhibited the growth of multiple strains of influenza A and B viruses in cell cultures.[44]

During a flu outbreak in an Israeli kibbutz, twenty-seven subjects were given either elderberry or a placebo for three days. The results were amazing: 90 percent of those who were given elderberry were entirely well after only three days. The others, who took the placebo, required six days to feel better.[45] I recommend a standardized extract of elderberry. Take two to four tablespoons daily of Black Elderberry Extract, or as directed by your physician.

Oscillococcinum

Oscillococcinum, the most popular over-the-counter flu treatment in France, has been used for over sixty years. Oscillococcinum is a homeopathic mixture containing a diluted extract of duck liver and heart and comes in granule form. Studies have shown that oscillococcinum may reduce the duration of the illness and severity of the symptoms. A study reported in the April 1998 issue of *British Homeopathic Journal* said 17.4 percent of those who took the supplement of oscillococcinum experienced no symptoms the following day compared with only 6 percent of those who took placebos.[46]

An article published in 2015 looked at several studies on the effectiveness of oscillococcinum; the studies did show an improvement in the symptoms of the flu in patients treated with oscillococcinum rather than a placebo.[47]

This remedy is to be used at the first sign of the flu, preferably within the first eight hours of symptoms, and can be found in most health food stores. Follow the instructions on the package for dosage.

Proteolytic enzymes

Proteolytic enzymes are anti-inflammatory agents that are extremely effective in treating sinusitis. Bromelain is a proteolytic enzyme found in pineapple juice and the stems of the pineapple plants.

In 1993 Germany's Commission E approved bromelain for reducing swelling of the nose and sinuses caused by injuries and operations.

A typical dosage of bromelain is 500 mg three times a day, taken between meals on an empty stomach.

Papaya and bromelain enzyme tablets also may help relieve sinus congestion and Eustachian tube blockage. Clear-ease is an enzyme product that contains bromelain and papaya enzymes. It actually contains one million enzyme units of bromelain and 500,000 units of papaya. It is recommended that you melt this in your mouth three times a day.

Phytosterols

One of the most important supplements in preventing colds, flu, and sinus infections is phytosterols. Sterols are plant fats that are similar to the animal fat cholesterol. All plants—including vegetables, fruits, nuts, and seeds—contain sterols and sterolins.

These sterols play a very important role in immune activity. Phytosterols can help T-cells multiply. In fact, one study showed T-cell response to this substance increasing from 20 percent to 920 percent after only four weeks on the sterol/sterolin mixture.

Another experiment showed dramatic increases in natural killer cell activity. I've found phytosterols very effective in protecting many individuals against developing colds, flu, and sinus infections.

You can obtain phytosterols in an over-the-counter product called Moducare. I recommend one tablet three times a day, one hour before meals, or two in the morning and one in the evening on an empty stomach.

Olive leaf extract

A bitter substance called *oleuropein* has been isolated from the olive leaf. The active ingredient in oleuropein has been found to possess powerful antibacterial properties as well as to inhibit the growth of viruses. The olive leaf has the ability to interrupt the replication of many different pathogens, including bacteria and viruses. It has been found to be effective in treating the flu, colds, and sinus infections.

The dose of this extract typically is 500 mg every six hours, taken between meals. For acute infections, some physicians recommend two tablets every six hours.

Silver biotic or active silver

You probably have heard the expression "He was born with a silver spoon in his mouth." It comes from the awful days of the plagues in Europe when no antibiotics or other medicines existed to stop the murderous rampage of disease that wiped out entire towns. Wealthier babies were given silver spoons to suck on throughout the day. The silver in the spoons provided an antibiotic effect, giving these infants a better chance at survival.

Today silver is still valued for its medicinal powers. Colloidal silver is a clear liquid composed of 99.9 percent pure silver particles, which are about 0.001–0.01 microns in diameter and are suspended in pure water. I do not recommend colloidal silver since it is associated with side effects including argyria, or a silver or gray discoloration of the skin. Colloidal silver typically contains 50,000–300,000 parts per million of silver. However, silver biotic, a new technology for silver, only contains 5 to 20 parts per million and will not cause argyria.

Silver biotic technology uses 10,000 volts of alternating current, whereas colloidal silver uses 110 volts of direct current. This increase in power supercharges the silver, giving it catalytic capabilities, destroying viruses, bacteria, and mold. Silver biotic can kill bacteria in only six minutes, and it can suppress and limit the effects of viral infections.[48] This silver biotic solution can be taken orally, sprayed in the nose as nasal spray, or nebulized and inhaled in the lungs or taken as a throat lozenge.

Xlear

Xlear contains xylitol, which is a naturally occurring sugar alcohol found in many fruits and vegetables that tastes and looks just like sugar.

This substance causes bacteria to lose their grip on the body's membranes, rendering them unable to grow. Once its hold is broken, xylitol then helps flush the harmful bacteria away.

Antibiotics tend to kill both good and bad bacteria, and they give rise to resistant bacteria growth. Xlear is an excellent treatment for sinus infections. It is also very safe to use in children.

Saventaro

Saventaro is a form of cat's claw, an herb used by the people in the Andes, especially in Peru, to treat ailments including infections, arthritis, dysentery, and inflammation. Cat's claw contains alkaloids that stimulate the immune system. Its active ingredient is a group of compounds called "pentacyclic oxindole alkaloids," also known as POAs.

Saventaro is the first and only form of cat's claw that comes from the root, where the POAs are far more concentrated. This makes this product much more potent than regular cat's claw.

- For colds, flu, and sinus infections, take two capsules three times a day for seven to ten days.

I also recommend that my patients use the Neti pot or SinuCleanse, available in most pharmacies over the counter. This uses a solution of saline and bicarbonate to flush out the nasal passages, relieving sinus infections, colds, and flus.

DIABETES

Both type 1 and type 2 diabetes can be helped by nutritional supplements. You must remember that supplements cannot take the place of a complete program to control and reverse type 2 diabetes that includes a focus on weight reduction, a good dietary plan, a regular exercise program, as well as stress reduction and hormone replacement therapy. Type 1 diabetics should *not* go off their insulin.

I recommend those with diabetes read *The New Bible Cure for Diabetes* and *Let Your Food Be Your Medicine* and follow the dietary recommendations in addition to using supplements.

Following is a complete list of nutrients and supplements that will help you fight type 2 diabetes. (If you have type 1 diabetes, these supplements are still helpful to your overall health; however, the supplements listed below that will be of greatest benefit in fighting your form of diabetes are alpha lipoic acid, vitamin D, chromium, PGX (short for PolyGlycopleX) fiber, omega 3, and the supplements for decreasing glycation.)

- **A good multivitamin**

The foundation of a good supplement program always starts with a good comprehensive multivitamin. Adequate doses of nutrients found in a good multivitamin include magnesium, chromium, vanadium, biotin and the B vitamins, and the macro minerals and trace minerals.

- Magnesium is essential for glucose balance and is important for the release of insulin and the maintenance of the pancreatic beta cells, which produce insulin. Magnesium also increases the affinity and number of insulin receptors, which are on the surface of cells. The recommended daily allowance for magnesium is 350 mg for men and 280 mg for women.

- Vanadium is another mineral that assists in the metabolism of glucose.
- Biotin is a B vitamin that helps prevent insulin resistance.

Even though a multivitamin is extremely important in forming the foundation of a nutritional supplement program, there are other key nutrients or a larger dose of certain vitamins and minerals that you need to take in addition to a good comprehensive multivitamin. Most physicians are unaware of which nutritional supplements are effective in lowering blood sugar levels. You will need to make your physician aware that you are taking supplements for diabetes. The supplements alone are able to lower one's blood sugar significantly, and diabetic medication dosages will usually eventually need to be lowered accordingly. When weight loss, regular exercise, my dietary program, stress reduction, and hormone replacement are combined with this list of nutritional supplements, the results are typically profound.

Vitamin D

Many Americans are not getting enough vitamin D, and we are beginning to see a close link between vitamin D deficiency and diabetes. According to a recent article published by researchers from Loyola University's Marcella Niehoff School of Nursing, vitamin D intake may prevent or delay the onset of diabetes as well as decrease complications for those who are diagnosed with diabetes. This article substantiated the role of vitamin D in the prevention as well as management of glucose intolerance and diabetes.[49]

Vitamin D also plays an important role in the secretion of insulin and in helping you avoid insulin resistance. Vitamin D not only decreases your blood sugar but also increases your body's sensitivity to insulin, thus making insulin more effective.

I check vitamin D levels on most of my patients by checking the 25-hydroxyvitamin D3 (25-OHD3) level. I typically try to get the patient's vitamin D level greater than fifty and less than eighty. I typically start most of my patients on 2,000 IU of vitamin D a day and may increase that amount to 4,000 IU or even 6,000 IU a day as I continue to monitor their 25-OHD3 level until the vitamin D level is greater than fifty. I then place them on a maintenance dose of vitamin D.

Chromium

Chromium is a mineral that is essential for good health. It has been of interest to diabetes researchers for a long time because it is required for normal metabolism of sugar, carbs, protein, and fat. Chromium is like insulin's little helper, and without adequate chromium, insulin cannot function properly.

How much chromium do you need? In 1989 the National Academy of

Sciences recommended an intake range for adults and adolescents of 50–200 mcg of chromium daily.[50] The Food and Nutrition Board of the Institute of Medicine has since narrowed this range down to 35 mcg for men and 25 mcg for women ages nineteen to fifty.[51]

A well-balanced diet should always be your first step in getting adequate amounts of vitamins, minerals, and other nutrients; however, fewer and fewer foods are providing the needed dietary intake levels of this important mineral. Whole grains and mushrooms may contain trace amounts of chromium, but that is only if these foods are grown in soils containing chromium. Likewise, seafood and some meat contain chromium, but only if the foods the animals ate contained chromium. Brewer's yeast is the only natural food source high in chromium; however, very few people eat this on a regular basis.

Also, the standard American diet, full of refined sugars and carbohydrates, actually *depletes* your body of chromium since these foods require chromium for metabolism. Type 2 diabetics in particular tend to be deficient in chromium, whether as a cause or result of their condition. I recommend type 2 diabetics avoid foods high in refined sugars and carbs and consider taking chromium in supplement form.

Be aware that chromium is commonly included in multivitamins, usually in amounts ranging from 100–200 mcg. For many people this may provide adequate supplementation.[52] Always inform your doctor before making any changes to your diet or supplement program; however, realize that most doctors are unaware of this information.

There are several forms of chromium used for supplementation, but the most common form is chromium picolinate. For my type 2 diabetic patients, I typically recommend supplementing chromium picolinate in the amount of 600–1,000 mcg a day in divided doses. One study conducted by Dr. Richard A. Anderson, PhD, formerly chief chemist at the USDA-ARS Nutrient Requirements and Functions Laboratory, found that type 2 diabetics who consumed 1,000 mcg per day of chromium improved insulin sensitivity without significant changes in body fat; type 1 diabetics were able to reduce their insulin dosage by 30 percent after only ten days of supplemental chromium picolinate at 200 mcg per day.[53]

Other studies in which researchers gave chromium to people with type 1 and type 2 diabetes have yielded mixed results. However, Dr. Anderson says that studies that show no beneficial effects using chromium for diabetes were usually using doses of chromium of 200 mcg or less, which is usually simply inadequate for diabetes, especially if the chromium is in the form that is poorly absorbed.[54]

Can you take too much chromium? According to Dr. Anderson's research, no discernible toxicity has been found in rats that consumed levels up to several thousand times the dietary reference for chromium for humans (based on body weight). There also have been no documented toxic effects in any of the human studies involving supplemental chromium, according to Dr. Anderson.[55] But again, please don't take massive amounts of any supplement without the advice of your doctor.

Alpha lipoic acid

Alpha lipoic acid is an important nutrient for fighting both type 1 and type 2 diabetes. Diabetics are more prone to oxidative stress and free-radical formation than nondiabetics. Lipoic acid is an amazing antioxidant that works in both water-soluble and fat-soluble compartments of the body and regenerates vitamin C, vitamin E, CoQ_{10}, and glutathione. Lipoic acid also improves insulin resistance in overweight adults suffering from type 2 diabetes.

Lipoic acid also can help relieve several components of metabolic syndrome: it can lower blood pressure, decrease insulin resistance, improve the lipid profile, and help individuals lose weight. Lipoic acid also has been used in Europe for decades to treat diabetic neuropathy with amazing success.

I usually start my diabetic patients on 600 mg of alpha lipoic acid two or three times a day, monitoring their blood sugars. Some patients develop gastrointestinal (GI) side effects, skin allergies, or decreased thyroid function, and I then decrease the dose to 200–300 mg two times per day. Scientific studies using doses ranging from 300–1,800 mg a day infer that the most important form of lipoic acid is R-dihydrolipoic acid, which is the most readily available form.[56] However, I find that alpha lipoic acid usually works best for the diabetic patients I have treated.

Soluble fiber

Good eating habits also help the battle against diabetes, particularly including soluble fiber in your diet. Soluble fiber not only helps slow the digestion of starches, but it also slows glucose uptake and thus lowers the glycemic index of your meal. This, in turn, lowers the amount of insulin that is secreted by the pancreas, which is very beneficial for those with type 2 diabetes. Soluble fiber also has been shown over the years through numerous studies to effectively lower blood sugar levels.[57]

How does it do all these things? Soluble fiber actually swells many times its original size as it binds to the water in your stomach and small intestine to form a glue-like gel that not only slows down the absorption of glucose but also induces a sense of satiety (fullness) and reduces your body's absorption of calories.

Studies conducted by James W. Anderson, MD, of the University of Kentucky, showed that high-fiber diets lowered insulin requirements an average of 38 percent in people with type 1 diabetes and 97 percent in people with type 2 diabetes. This means that almost all the people suffering from type 2 diabetes who followed Dr. Anderson's high-fiber diet were able to lower or stop taking insulin and other diabetes medications and still maintain a healthy blood sugar level. Additionally, these results lasted up to fifteen years.[58]

Fruit, beans, chickpeas, lentils, carrots, squash, oat bran, barley, rice bran, guar gum, glucomannan, and pectin are all very good sources of soluble fiber.

Supplementing with PGX

In addition to dietary sources of fiber, it's a good idea to supplement. I recommend a specific fiber supplement developed by scientists at the University of Toronto called PGX. Often called the new "super fiber," PGX is a unique blend of plant fibers containing glucomannan, a soluble and fermentable fiber derived from the root of the konjac plant. It also contains sodium alginate, xanthan gum, and mulberry leaf extract. It works the same as dietary sources of fiber; however, the specific ratio of natural compounds used in PGX enables it to be three to five times as effective as other fibers alone.

Clinical studies by Dr. Vuksan, the developer of PGX, have shown repeatedly that blood sugar levels after meals decrease as soluble fiber viscosity increases.[59] The exciting news is that PGX fiber lowers after-meal blood sugars by approximately 20 percent and also lowers insulin secretion by approximately 40 percent. This is unequaled by any drug or natural health-food product.

Recently researchers at the University of Toronto found that higher doses of PGX can decrease appetite significantly because PGX absorbs six hundred times its weight in water over one to two hours and expands in the digestive tract.[60]

Most soluble fiber has side effects of producing significant amounts of gas; however, PGX has fewer GI side effects than other dietary fiber, mainly because PGX can be given in much smaller quantities than other viscous fibers and achieve comparable health benefits without all the gas.

Anytime you increase your fiber intake, you should start slowly and drink plenty of water. With PGX, I recommend that you start with one capsule, three times a day, before meals, with sixteen ounces of water, and gradually increase the dose as tolerated every two to three days. Most people use two to three softgels before meals with sixteen ounces of water. Rarely will someone need six softgels before meals, which is the maximum dose.

Cinnamon

Studies have shown that cinnamon may help lower blood sugar levels as well as cholesterol for those with type 2 diabetes. One study conducted showed that even 1 g of cinnamon taken daily for forty days reduced blood glucose and cholesterol levels in both men and women with type 2 diabetes.[61] Cinnamon can be added to food as well as taken as a supplement.

Omega-3 fatty acids

Omega-3 fats are simply polyunsaturated fats that come from foods such as fish, fish oil, vegetable oils (especially flaxseed oil), walnuts, and wheat germ. However, the most beneficial omega-3 fats are fish oils containing eicosapentaenoic acid (EPA) and docosahexaenoic acid (DHA).

Omega-3 fats generally protect against heart disease, decrease inflammation, lower triglyceride levels, and may help prevent insulin resistance and improve glucose tolerance. Fish oil also helps decrease the rate of developing diabetic vascular complications.

Dietary fats that are considered to be beneficial include not only fish oils but also avocados, extra-virgin olive oil, almond butter, nuts, and seeds. A word of caution: some fish oil supplements may contain mercury, pesticides, or polychlorinated biphenyls (PCBs).

I usually place my patients with prediabetes and those with diabetes on 320–1,000 mg of fish oils three times a day. If they have high triglyceride levels, I may increase the dose to 4,000–5,000 mg a day. Caution: fish oil supplements may thin the blood and should not be used with blood thinners unless recommended by one's physician.

Carnosine

Glycation is the name for protein molecules that bind to glucose molecules and form advanced glycation end products (AGEs). Glycated proteins produce fifty times more free radicals than nonglycated proteins. Typical manifestations of this are skin wrinkling and brain degeneration. Both prediabetics and diabetics are much more prone to glycation and, as a result, will age prematurely.

The amino acid carnosine, however, helps stabilize and protect cell membranes from glycation. Carnosine is a safe and effective nutrient for inhibiting glycation. I usually recommend at least 1,000 mg a day of carnosine to my diabetic patients.

Environmental Allergies

If you sneeze, wheeze, cough and drain, and have weepy eyes because of airborne allergens, the following list of vitamins and supplements usually will help your symptoms.

Bioflavonoids

Bioflavonoids are also effective against allergy symptoms. They are potent anti-inflammatories and are found in the white pith of citrus fruits and other foods containing vitamin C. Bioflavonoids boost the immune system and help limit histamine reactions. You can find them in vitamin and mineral supplements such as vitamin C with bioflavonoids.

Grape seed extract

Grape seed extract is another bioflavonoid that, taken with vitamin C, helps suppress allergic reactions. I recommend a dose between 100 mg and 300 mg a day.

Omega-3 fatty acid

This is fish oil. A dose of approximately one or two 1,000-mg capsules taken at each meal may help protect against allergic attacks. Caution: consult your physician if taking aspirin or blood thinners since this dose may thin the blood.

Pantothenic acid

Pantothenic acid, or vitamin B_5, helps support both the adrenals and thymus gland, which will, in turn, minimize allergic responses. Take a dose of 300–500 mg per day. As you take supplements to support the adrenal glands, allergies usually improve.

Quercetin

Quercetin is a bioflavonoid that reduces histamine levels. Take quercetin in a dose of 500 mg two to three times a day, along with buffered vitamin C, to relieve allergy symptoms. Quercetin also is found in yellow and red onions.

Vitamin C

I recommend 500–1,000 mg of buffered vitamin C two to three times a day. High levels of buffered vitamin C in the body have an antihistamine effect. Vitamin C also helps support the adrenal glands.

My favorite supplement for environmental allergies is Healthy Sinus Formula (see appendix A).

As you are faithful to take these vitamins and supplements, you will strengthen your immune system and help your body fight off allergy symptoms to any environmental allergens you may encounter.

Food Allergies and Sensitivities

Food allergies and sensitivities are a typical inflammatory response triggered by foods. The most common food allergies are caused by eggs, cow's milk and other dairy products, peanuts, wheat (gluten), soy, tree nuts (such as almonds, cashews, pecans, or walnuts), fish, shellfish, and seeds (sesame and sunflower seeds). An estimated forty to fifty million Americans have environmental allergies, but only about 4 percent of all adults are allergic to foods or food additives. Among children under the age of four, this increases to 7 percent.[62] The percent of people with food sensitivity is much higher than food allergies. Refer to appendix A for information on the antigen leukocyte cellular antibody test (ALCAT) to identify your food sensitivities.

Refer to my book *Let Food Be Your Medicine,* follow the anti-inflammation Mediterranean diet, and rotate your foods.

If you are experiencing food allergies, and as a result are suffering gastrointestinal problems, there are plenty of vitamins and supplements that can help you restore your intestinal health.

Deglycyrrhizinated licorice (DGL)

I recommend DGL. DGL is a form of licorice that has had glycyrrhetinic acid removed, since glycyrrhetinic acid occasionally causes high blood pressure. DGL helps to restore the cells of the stomach and small intestines. You can find it at your local health food store. Chew one to two tablets before meals. The typical dose is 300–400 mg of DGL one to three times a day.

Glutamine

To heal the cells of the small intestines and to repair impaired intestinal permeability, I recommend one to two tablets, or 500–1,000 mg, of glutamine two or three times a day. Take them about thirty minutes before each meal.

Probiotics

Probiotics are beneficial bacteria that reside in the GI tract. Having an abundance of different probiotics in the GI tract contribute greatly to a healthy GI tract and prevention of food allergies. I also recommend one tablespoon of chia seeds in eight ounces of water two times a day since this serves as food for the beneficial bacteria and provides both soluble and insoluble fiber.

A recent study found that clostridia, a type of gut bacteria, may help limit food allergies. The theory is that our lifestyle, including the abundance of antibiotic use and the foods we eat, has changed the bacteria in our guts. Studies have shown an improvement when this bacteria was introduced in mice.[63]

Headaches

Often those who are suffering from migraines and tension headaches are significantly depleted in certain vitamins and minerals. Other herbs and supplements can dramatically reduce headache symptoms. Let's take a closer look at these natural marvels and see how they can help you find healing from headaches.

In addition to supplements, follow an anti-inflammatory diet, and if your headaches are not improving within a few months, I recommend the antigen leukocyte cellular antibody test (ALCAT) to see which foods may be triggering your headaches.

- **Magnesium**

This is an essential mineral that maintains the tone of blood vessels. Many migraine sufferers do not have enough magnesium. You can find out if your body is lacking magnesium by asking your doctor to check an erythrocyte magnesium level. A serum magnesium level is not as reliable as an erythrocyte magnesium level because it does not always indicate tissue levels of magnesium, and therefore it is less helpful.

Magnesium citrate and aspartate are chelated forms of magnesium, which are absorbed better than most other forms. I recommend approximately 200–250 mg two to three times a day. However, start with only one tablet a day since magnesium can cause diarrhea.

Fish oil

Supplement your diet with one to two fish oil capsules (1,000 mg) twice a day. Fish oil supplies essential fatty acids that decrease arachidonic acid, a dangerous form of fat that may trigger migraines.

Feverfew

Feverfew is an herb that both prevents and relieves migraine headaches for many individuals. Feverfew inhibits the release of vasodilating substances from platelets and thus helps maintain blood vessel tone. The active ingredient in feverfew is parthenolide (which is listed on the label). Take feverfew with 0.5 mg of parthenolide per day.

Feverfew has been used as a migraine remedy for over two centuries. A 1988 British study revealed that daily intake of only 82 mg of feverfew over four months led to fewer headaches, and the headaches that did occur were much milder.[64]

5-hydroxytryptophan (5-HTP)

5-HTP is an amino acid that is very useful in preventing migraine headaches by increasing the levels of serotonin and endorphins in the brain. 5-HTP also helps relieve depression and stress, which are common migraine triggers. I recommend 50–100 mg of 5-HTP three times a day, with each meal. If you are taking an antidepressant or a migraine medication such as Imitrex, consult your doctor before taking 5-HTP. You also may take 150–300 mg of 5-HTP at bedtime to raise your serotonin levels and prevent sleep-induced migraines. Do not take over 450 mg of 5-HTP a day unless your nutritional doctor recommends it.

Riboflavin (vitamin B_2)

Riboflavin, when taken in fairly large doses on a daily basis, has been shown to reduce the number of migraine headaches in individuals. A study found that 400 mg of riboflavin a day was very effective in preventing migraine headaches, reducing migraines from four days a month to two days a month after three to six months.[65]

Butterbur (Petadolex)

Supplementing with butterbur, taken by mouth, may help prevent migraine headaches as well as lowering their intensity and the length of time they last. It is thought that butterbur is effective because it limits the body's inflammation and spasms, which are both contributing factors to migraines. In one study a dose of butterbur 75 mg two times a day was associated with a migraine frequency reduction of 48 percent.[66]

Water

Water is the most important nutrient for migraines. I have found many of my migraine patients are mildly to moderately dehydrated, and drinking water throughout the day often prevents migraines. I recommend alkaline water and have my patients follow my alkaline instructions: stay away from caffeine, alcohol, chocolate, citrus fruits, spicy food, onions, garlic, and tomatoes. It's also important to adjust the urine pH to 7.0–7.5. Most migraine sufferers have an acidic urine pH, which causes the body to lose valuable minerals, including magnesium and calcium.

Heart Disease

While congestive heart failure is very serious and certain arrhythmias (abnormality in the heartbeat) could lead to sudden death, they are typically both very treatable. As with most muscles in the body, the heart can be maintained and even strengthened. Treatment is all about reenergizing and refueling the heart by increasing blood flow to it and supplying nutrients to strengthen the heart and give it more energy. You might think of it like recharging the "battery cells" of the heart. It is really a question of getting as much "energy" generated for the heart as possible.

As with any other muscle, this energy starts at the cellular level, and the powerhouse of the cell is mitochondria, small organelles inside each cell that generate energy by synthesizing fuel (food) and oxygen and making adenosine triphosphate (ATP). Mitochondria generate over 90 percent of the energy the body uses and make up about 35 percent of heart cells. It is mitochondrial energy that drives the metabolism. ATP is the heart's energy currency. Mitochondrial energy is produced in a process that uses oxygen and nutrients to change ATP into adenosine diphosphate (ADP) and inorganic phosphate (Pi), then changes those two back to ATP again. This cycle is almost like the turning of a turbine, releasing energy with each change. If the cell is deficient in fuel or oxygen, this cycle suffers; thus the cell's metabolism suffers and its function is compromised.

The by-product of this cycle is carbon dioxide (CO_2), water, and a small amount of damaged oxygen molecules that are missing an electron—in other words, free radicals. The CO_2 is exhaled when we breathe, along with a little of the water, while the rest of the water travels to the kidneys. If the free radicals accumulate to high levels, it can cause problems; however, there is evidence that some level of them may be important for functions such as mitochondrial respiration, white blood cell activity, and platelet activation. Very high levels, though, will injure the cell membranes, degrade the mitochondria and other parts of the cell, as well as damage DNA. To prevent this, I recommend glutathione-boosting supplements, which is the body's most important antioxidant.

The key to optimizing this energy-producing cycle is keeping the mitochondria healthy. If we have healthy mitochondria, then most likely we will be healthy too. Healthy mitochondria protect against any number of degenerative diseases, such as cardiovascular disease, cancer, and Alzheimer's disease.

Nutrients for a healthy heart muscle

Consider taking these supplements to improve the health of your heart.

RiboCeine or N-acetyl cysteine

RiboCeine is a blend of D-ribose and L-Cysteine, and it is the most powerful glutathione-boosting supplement available. Glutathione is the most important antioxidant in the body, and boosting it is important for heart health. Glutathione is necessary to fight free radicals, and it also helps repair and recycle other antioxidants in your body. RiboCeine is the best way to boost glutathione. I recommend MaxOne (RiboCeine) one capsule twice a day or N-acetyl cysteine 500 mg to 1000 mg capsule twice a day.

Coenzyme Q_{10} (CoQ_{10})

The antioxidant CoQ_{10} functions as a coenzyme in the energy-producing pathways of every cell in the body and is an important antioxidant that will fight the oxidation that creates free radicals as well as the oxidation of low-density lipoprotein (LDL) and other lipids. CoQ_{10}'s most important function is probably within the mitochondria that facilitate the productivity of ATP, which is so crucial to the health of every cell and particularly important in the cells of the heart muscle.

When you take CoQ_{10} as a supplement, pay attention to what form it comes in. Research has shown that since it is such a large molecule, it is hard to absorb. The best form to take it in is ubiquinol, which is the active form. As many as 30 percent of Japanese have a defective NADH quinone oxidoreductase 1 (NQO1) gene that regulates CoQ_{10} from the inactive ubiquinone to the active ubiquinol. Also, as you age, the conversion process slows down.

For basic health, I recommend 100 mg of ubiquinol a day. For congestive heart failure (CHF), I recommend 200 mg of ubiquinol two to three times a day, and for severe CHF, you may need 200–400 mg of ubiquinol two to three times a day. If you are taking a statin drug, I recommend 100–300 mg a day of ubiquinol. I also check the CoQ_{10} blood level and adjust the dose accordingly. Life Extension performs this blood test.

Pyrroloquinoline quinone (PQQ)

PQQ is a supplement that helps resuscitate the mitochondria. Low or dysfunctional mitochondria is a mark of many diseases, including heart disease or heart failure. PQQ is an antioxidant that is emerging as the micronutrient that may reverse cellular aging. It plays an essential role in defending cells against mitochondrial decay. It helps with this by participating "in the energy transfer within the mitochondria that supplies the body with most of its bioenergy," as a *Life Extension* article reports.[67] PQQ's chemical structure enables it to withstand exposure to oxidation up to five thousand times greater than vitamin C. It not only protects mitochondria from damage, but it also stimulates growth of new mitochondria.

L-carnitine

Another "transport" molecule that helps in mitochondrial energy generation is L-carnitine, which facilitates moving long-chain fatty acids across the inner mitochondrial membrane to catalyze beta-oxidation, a process by which the fat is broken down so it can be burned as fuel and turned into energy. L-carnitine is one of the most easily used amino acids in our bodies and is also a precursor of nitric oxide and other metabolites. These fatty acids must be brought through the mitochondrial membrane to be processed in this way, and L-carnitine is the only carrier molecule that can do this. Thus the higher the level of L-carnitine in your system, the greater the rate of energy metabolism, and the lower the level, the more difficult it is to generate sufficient energy. Since the heart gets at least 60 percent of its fuel from such fat sources, L-carnitine is crucial to heart health and improving congestive heart failure.

- L-carnitine is found in protein-rich foods such as peanuts, Brazil nuts, walnuts, coconut, milk and milk products, pork, beef, chicken, turkey, seafood, oats, wheat, and chocolate. However, with age, through genetic defects, or eating carnitine-deficient diets (as pure vegetarians often do), deficiencies of other vitamins and minerals important to L-carnitine, liver or kidney disease, and the use of certain prescription drugs are all associated with our bodies having insufficient levels of L-carnitine; therefore, supplementation is vital. L-carnitine should be supplemented in a dose of 500 mg three times a day. For severe CHF, I usually increase the dose to 1,000 mg three times a day.

D-ribose

This is a simple five-carbon sugar found in every cell of the body. It is different from other sugars, such as glucose (a six-carbon sugar) because it both provides and sustains energy, especially in weakened hearts. D-ribose provides tremendous support to the mitochondria in assisting the mitochondria to produce ATP, or the heart's energy currency.

D-ribose is naturally present in some meats, but only in trace amounts so small it does not really make any meaningful impact on our bodies. Cells synthesize D-ribose as they need it to varying degrees, but supplementation of D-ribose is the best way to provide it within your body because it is easily absorbed.

I recommend the following daily dosages for the following concerns:

- As a daily preventative of cardiovascular disease or for those who exercise strenuously on a regular basis: 5–7 g a day (5 g is equivalent to two teaspoons)
- For someone with mild to moderate congestive heart failure, recovering from a heart attack or heart surgery, or those with other significant vascular concerns or as a treatment for angina: 7–10 g a day in divided doses
- For advanced congestive heart failure, dilated cardiomyopathy, frequent angina, and those awaiting heart transplants or suffering from severe fibromyalgia: 10–15 g a day in divided doses

Magnesium

Magnesium is a wonderful mineral for the heart and cardiovascular system across the board. If you're suffering with congestive heart failure or arrhythmia, magnesium may be a significant help to you. In fact, magnesium deficiency is very common in those who have congestive heart failure. Studies show that as many as half of Americans lack the magnesium they should have, oddly enough roughly the same number who have cardiovascular complications.

Magnesium is present in nuts, grains, beans, and dark green vegetables. Alcohol and caffeine consumption encourage the excretion of magnesium. Certain conventional drugs for treating congestive heart failure, such as Lanoxin and various diuretics, also may deplete magnesium levels.

Most individuals who have experienced congestive heart failure should take a magnesium supplement. It is also beneficial in treating arrhythmia, including atrial fibrillation, premature ventricular contractions (PVCs), and symptoms of mitral valve prolapse. I recommend a dose of 200 mg two to three times a day. Use caution with magnesium since it may cause diarrhea. Start with 200 mg two times a day, and increase very slowly if needed.

CHF treatments

Testosterone

Testosterone supplementation is also very important for all people with CHF. There are more testosterone receptors in cardiac muscle than any other muscle in the body. Testosterone also will help strengthen the heart muscle. I even place women with CHF on a low dose of testosterone, usually with 1–5 mg of transdermal testosterone once a day. Heavy metal detoxification, chelation therapy, and an infrared sauna also may be very important for people with CHF. People with CHF sometimes have high mercury, lead, and/or cadmium levels in their cardiac muscle, and the heavy metals may be poisoning their mitochondria or their energy-producing structures in the cell.

Arrhythmia treatments

The above supplements not only help CHF but also help arrhythmia. An arrhythmia is any change in the regular rhythm of the heart. It is typically due to interference with the electrical pathways of the heart and is responsible for over 400,000 deaths each year. Some arrhythmias are harmless, and some are life threatening. Often the first sign of hidden heart disease is sudden death, which is usually caused by arrhythmias. If you have an arrhythmia, consider getting a sleep study to rule out sleep apnea. Sleep apnea is associated with lower oxygen levels in the body and arrhythmias. Here are other supplements that usually help:

Omega-3 fats

Omega-3 fats from fish oil may prevent sudden death. The Italian Gruppo Italiano per lo Studio della Streptochinasi nell'Infarto Miocardico (GISSI-Prevenzione) was a trial of over eleven thousand participants who either took 1,000 mg of EPA and DHA (fish oil) or a placebo. The group taking fish oil had a 30 percent reduction in cardiovascular mortality and a 45 percent reduction in sudden death.[68] A Harvard study showed that men who had higher blood levels of omega-3 fats had an 80 percent lower risk of sudden death compared with men with low serum levels of omega-3.[69] Omega-3 fats also may help prevent atrial fibrillation. I recommend 1,000 mg of EPA/DHA two to four times a day. (Consult your doctor if you are taking blood thinners.)

Magnesium

Magnesium deficiency is associated with arrhythmias including atrial fibrillation and atrial flutter. Atrial fibrillation is the most common sustained arrhythmia. Magnesium strongly impacts heart cell membrane function and is a very important catalyst in many enzymatic reactions in the heart muscle cell (myocyte) and in more than three hundred enzymatic reactions in the body. Magnesium given intravenously also has been shown to reduce the frequency of ventricular arrhythmias in patients with symptomatic heart failure. Magnesium helps prevent both benign arrhythmias and serious arrhythmias.

Magnesium helps relax the heart and calm down and stabilize the heart's electrical system. I typically recommend 200 mg of chelated magnesium two to three times a day. Start with a low dose, and increase slowly to prevent diarrhea.

Taurine

Taurine is the second most abundant amino acid in muscle. Foods that contain taurine include meat, poultry, eggs, dairy, and fish. Taurine prevents arrhythmias by limiting calcium overload of the myocardium and helping to prevent hypertrophy of the heart. The heart that is ischemic, or lacking adequate oxygen, is more prone to arrhythmia. Some researchers believe that arrhythmias due to acute myocardial ischemia may be due to a loss of intracellular taurine. Following either an ischemic event or heart attack, taurine levels drop to as low as one-third of normal levels. Taurine also protects the oxygen-starved, or ischemic, heart from reperfusion-induced arrhythmias. I recommend at least 500–1,000 mg twice a day; however, doses up to 6,000 mg a day have been used in some studies.

Coenzyme Q_{10} (ubiquinol)

I have already discussed CoQ_{10} in detail; however, it is also very useful in treating arrhythmias. CoQ_{10} is found in every cell of the body and helps manufacture energy. It also is believed to stabilize the heart's electrical system and help prevent arrhythmias. It is especially effective for premature ventricular contractions (PVCs). I usually recommend ubiquinol in a daily dose of 100–300 mg or more a day.

Berberine

Berberine is the main active ingredient in the herb goldenseal, which has been used for years to treat intestinal infections. It also has been found to be beneficial for ventricular arrhythmias due to ischemia, or a lack of oxygen. Berberine also may help prevent sudden death after myocardial ischemic damage.

Researchers have studied berberine in patients with ventricular arrhythmias. They found that 62 percent of patients had 50 percent or greater, and 38 percent of patients had 90 percent or greater suppression of PVCs. Berberine is typically recommended at a dose of 500 mg twice a day.

Most all supplements that help congestive heart failure and ischemia will also typically help arrhythmias. The herb hawthorn also may help control benign arrhythmias in a dose of 80–300 mg twice a day.

Heartburn

It is important to remove several triggers of heartburn. These include caffeine, alcohol, nicotine, chocolate, citrus fruits, spicy food, onions, garlic, tomatoes, mint (including peppermint and spearmint), and fatty and fried foods. Some other tips include watching your weight, not overeating, avoiding eating before sleeping, avoiding exercise too soon after eating, and elevating the head of your bed thirty degrees or more. Also eat your food slowly, chewing every bit thirty times, and limit your beverage to only eight ounces with meals.

Supplements also may be helpful in the treatment of heartburn. Consider taking these supplements.

Deglycyrrhizinated licorice (DGL)

Deglycyrrhizinated licorice, also known as DGL, has been shown to soothe the digestive tract and stomach lining. It also may be effective against H. pylori, a bacteria in the stomach that is associated with ulcers and gastritis. Research has shown this also can help with heartburn. Make sure you take DGL rather than another licorice compound because it does not contain glycyrrhizin, which can cause health problems in high doses.[70] The dose of DGL is typically 300–400 mg one to three times a day.

D-limonene

This supplement, which comes from the rinds of citrus fruits, has been shown to relieve symptoms of heartburn in many patients. Two small studies were done, so further study is needed. However, the results so far are promising; in the first study, participants were given the supplement every other day and discontinued their medication. Two weeks later, 89 percent were symptom free. In the second, participants were given either the supplement or a placebo. Eighty-six percent of those taking the supplement were symptom free two weeks later, as opposed to 29 percent of those taking the placebo.[71] There is some evidence that taking D-limonene for just twenty days may relieve symptoms for up to six months. It is thought that this supplement coats the esophagus with a protective layer that eliminates pain from acid reflux. It also may lower the amount of acid that goes up into the esophagus. Take one 1,000 mg capsule every other day for twenty days. After that time period, you may occasionally take one capsule as needed.[72]

Mastic gum

Mastic gum is made from the sap of the mastic tree. It reduces symptoms of heartburn as well as other gastrointestinal issues, such as ulcers and gastritis. It is thought that this supplement reduces the amount of stomach acid, and it also may protect the stomach from acid.[73] Take 250–500 mg two times a day on an empty stomach for heartburn. I usually recommend a product that contains both mastic gum and DGL. (See appendix A.)

HEPATITIS AND HEPATITIS C

Hepatitis A is called "infectious hepatitis" because the virus spreads through contaminated food and water. This type of hepatitis is very common in third-world countries. Most of those who contract it recover their health. Victims of hepatitis A do not develop chronic infections.

Hepatitis B is a little different. It is called "serum hepatitis" because it is transmitted to others through blood and other body fluids. Most adults—95 percent—recover from hepatitis B, though a small percentage develop a chronic infection. Of the nearly 200,000 people who are infected by hepatitis B each year, only about 10,000 develop a chronic hepatitis B infection.

Hepatitis C was discovered relatively recently and was first called the hepatitis C virus in 1989. Before this it was simply known as non-A, non-B hepatitis. Testing for both hepatitis A and B was possible in the 1960s and 1970s. But blood tests to identify hepatitis C were not developed until 1990.

Hepatitis C is the most common chronic infection transmitted by the blood in the United States. However, unlike hepatitis B, of those who contract hepatitis C, only 15 percent actually recover. Worldwide, nearly 150 million individuals suffer with chronic hepatitis C.

Building up your body's immune system so that it has the strength it needs to win its battle against hepatitis C requires godly wisdom. If you or a loved one has hepatitis C, strengthening your body will require making wise nutritional choices. But that is not all. Your immune system is waging a long battle and needs incredible resources to endure and overcome. That's why adding nutritional supplements can make a vital difference for you. Supplements will provide your body with the vital resources it needs to give it strength and endurance to meet and beat the challenge it is facing.

The supplements we will discuss are recommended for all stages of hepatitis C except cirrhosis of the liver. People suffering from cirrhosis must be closely monitored by their physician, and supplements may need to be reduced according to their doctor's recommendations.

Get a good multivitamin

Patients with hepatitis C must avoid vitamin and mineral deficiencies since this will directly affect the immune system and may accelerate the disease process, leading to fibrosis, cirrhosis of the liver, and even liver cancer.

Always start your supplement program with a good comprehensive multivitamin/mineral supplement. A comprehensive multivitamin, such as Divine Health's Enhanced Multivitamin, is absolutely essential for the health of all patients with hepatitis C. A good multivitamin should contain at least 400 IU of vitamin E, 400 IU of vitamin D, 100–200 mcg of selenium, all eight of the B vitamins, vitamin C, and zinc. The mineral selenium is especially important for patients with hepatitis C.

Taking a comprehensive multivitamin and mineral supplement will help your body get enough vitamins, minerals, and antioxidants every day. It will give your immune system most of the raw materials it requires to do its job well.

Cautions for these supplements

A good multivitamin/mineral formula provides a foundation for your supplementation program, giving you the balance of nutrients that you need. But it is important to understand that excessive amounts of certain vitamins and minerals can actually be dangerous to your liver. You should be aware of the following cautions regarding these supplements.

Vitamin A

Too much vitamin A can damage the liver. For that reason, I do not recommend taking over 10,000 IU of vitamin A per day.

Niacin

Another vitamin that is potentially toxic to the liver when taken in high doses is niacin. Doses of 20–100 mg of niacin per day is usually sufficient. However, to lower cholesterol, many doctors prescribe doses of 500–1,000 mg of niacin two to three times per day. This can be toxic to a patient with hepatitis C. If you are taking niacin because of elevated cholesterol, be sure and have your liver functions checked after the first month and then at least every three to four months thereafter. Because high doses of niacin may cause inflammation of the liver, patients with hepatitis C should be monitored more closely.

Iron

If you have hepatitis C, you should not take any supplemental iron unless your doctor advises it. The hepatitis C virus actually needs iron to thrive. That's why patients with high iron levels are more prone to experience the progression of hepatitis C to fibrosis, cirrhosis, and even liver cancer.

So never supplement with a multivitamin tablet that contains iron, and never take supplemental iron if you have hepatitis C. This is another reason why you should dramatically decrease your consumption of red meat to three to six ounces only one time a week or less frequently.

Antioxidant support

The following supplements are antioxidants that may be helpful for those with hepatitis, particularly those with hepatitis C.

Vitamin C

High doses of vitamin C have antiviral qualities that have been known to help some individuals with hepatitis C. However, one caution when considering a higher dose of vitamin C is that it may cause increased uptake of iron from the gastrointestinal tract. In other words, it can help your body absorb even more iron from your food. We mentioned that iron promotes the disease process for hepatitis C. If you take high doses of vitamin C (over 1,000 mg a day), be sure to have your serum iron and ferritin levels checked by your physician if you have hepatitis C.

Alpha lipoic acid

One of the best supplements you can take for protecting the liver is alpha lipoic acid. This powerful antioxidant does its work of fighting and extinguishing free radicals, which cause a great deal of damage at the cellular level.

Some antioxidants are only effective in certain areas of the body where they can be absorbed, such as fat-soluble or water-soluble tissues. However, alpha lipoic acid is powerfully effective in tissues throughout the body. In addition to that, it helps the body produce glutathione, which is another powerful antioxidant that protects liver cells and destroys viruses.

Alpha lipoic acid is the only antioxidant that can recycle or renew itself as well as recycle other antioxidants, including vitamin E, vitamin C, CoQ_{10}, and glutathione.[74]

These are some of the powerful effects alpha lipoic acid has on the body:

- It helps protect the liver.
- It aids in regenerating the liver.
- It stimulates the immune system.
- It reduces the risk of developing cirrhosis and liver cancer.

With all these incredible benefits, it's easy to see why this supplement is considered by some to be the most important supplement for hepatitis C.

I recommend taking 300–600 mg of alpha lipoic acid two to three times a day.

Amino acids

Amino acids also can help those with hepatitis C. Consider taking the following supplements.

N-acetyl cysteine (NAC)

One of the most important amino acids that you can take for your liver is N-acetyl cysteine, otherwise known as NAC. NAC is hepatoprotective, which means it is a liver protector. In addition to that, it acts as a powerful antioxidant.

Supplementing with NAC enables your body to make its own glutathione, the powerful antioxidant that protects the liver. In other words, it is a "precursor" of glutathione. Some feel the key to its special liver protection qualities is its ability to increase the levels of glutathione within liver cells.

I recommend two 500-mg capsules of NAC twice a day, taken with food.

RiboCeine

RiboCeine is the most powerful glutathione-boosting supplement available—much more powerful than NAC. Boosting it is important for overall health, particularly for those with hepatitis. RiboCeine is the best way to boost glutathione. I recommend RiboCeine, one or two capsules twice a day. (See appendix A.)

S-adenosyl methionine (SAM-e)

SAM-e is an amino acid that helps prevent a fatty liver. A fatty liver is usually associated with alcoholism, obesity, or diabetes and involves fatty changes in the liver cells from fat deposits in the cells. A fatty liver also may cause inflammation of the liver.

SAM-e is useful as well in treating depression, which commonly accompanies hepatitis C. If your liver does not have enough of its own SAM-e, it cannot eliminate the amino acid methionine, which can build up to toxic levels.

If you are experiencing depression and have hepatitis C, I recommend taking 400 mg of SAM-e (one or two tablets) twice a day on an empty stomach.

Healing herbs

In addition to these supplements that can dramatically benefit your body in its battle against hepatitis C, a number of healing herbs can make a real difference. Here are some herbs that you can add to your supplement program in your battle against this disease.

Milk thistle

I personally believe the most important herb to use in the treatment of hepatitis C is milk thistle. Milk thistle contains a substance called silymarin, which blocks the formation of leukotrienes (substances in your cells involved in inflammation that damage your liver's cells). Silymarin helps your damaged liver regenerate liver tissue, as well as protects your liver from the damaging effects of the hepatitis virus.

That's not all. This powerful substance also goes to work acting as an antioxidant and quenching free-radical damage. It also is believed to help prevent glutathione deficiency in the liver cells.

Milk thistle may well be the most powerful herb for both protecting the liver against toxins that damage it and repairing damaged liver tissue. Taking milk thistle commonly improves liver function tests, especially the alanine aminotransferase (ALT) test.

I recommend taking 200 mg of milk thistle three times a day.

Other helpful herbs

Burdock root, schisandra chinensis, reishi mushrooms, Chinese bupleurum, picrorhiza, dandelion root, and aloe vera also may help patients with hepatitis C. However, prior to taking these herbs, consult a nutritional doctor, and continue to have your liver enzymes checked periodically.

Start with a comprehensive multivitamin, RiboCeine, lipoic acid, and milk thistle.

Don't take these herbs!

Never take herbs indiscriminately. Not all herbs are good for your liver, especially if you have hepatitis C. Some herbs can be very toxic and could cause harm. Here's a list of herbs to avoid if you have hepatitis C:

- Chaparral
- Mistletoe
- Germander
- Mate tea
- Hops
- Valerian
- Comfrey root
- Kava
- Yohimbe
- Skullcap

Caution: If you plan to take Chinese or American herbs as a part of your treatment for hepatitis C, it's very important to have your liver functions checked one month after beginning herbs and every three to four months thereafter. Immediately discontinue use of any herbs that cause an elevation in liver functions.

Finding a therapy that is right for you

There are many pathways to healing hepatitis C. Nutrition, supplements, herbs, medications, and prayer can all work together in concert in helping you to overcome this disease. There are also new conventional medical treatments for hepatitis C.

The best medicine for hepatitis C is Harvoni. Different combinations of drugs for hepatitis C have cure rates up to 100 percent, with a cure defined as having none of the virus in your body six months after treatment is complete.[75] These medications are very expensive but are very beneficial. I tell my patients that they should try to get their insurance to cover one of these medicines but in the meantime to follow my nutrition program for hepatitis C here or also found in *The Bible Cure for Hepatitis and Hepatitis C*.

High Cholesterol

In the section on diabetes I discussed how foods that are high in soluble fiber can reduce blood sugar. Fiber also can help reduce low-density lipoprotein (LDL) or bad cholesterol levels, as studies have shown. In a study, different types of soluble fiber were tested to see their effect on blood lipids. Decreases in cholesterol were small but significant.[76] Foods such as chia seeds, ground flaxseed, and psyllium seeds are inexpensive, a good source of fiber, and effective at lowering cholesterol. Chia seeds may be taken without grinding, and I typically recommend one tablespoon of chia seeds two to three times per day. Both flaxseed and psyllium seeds need to be ground, and the dose for them is one to three tablespoons two times per day. However, many people may find it difficult to take time to either prepare these kinds of foods or eat enough of them. For these individuals, I recommend soluble-fiber supplements such as PGX Fiber.

Choosing a fiber supplement

Over-the-counter fiber supplement products such as Metamucil contain psyllium husks, which are an excellent source of fiber. However, many of the liquid forms of these supplements contain sugar or NutraSweet, so be sure to read the labels.

Other forms of soluble fiber can be added to smoothies or mixed in cereals or oatmeal. These include oat bran, rice bran, psyllium seed, psyllium husks, guar gum, chia seeds, and flaxseed. I now use one tablespoon of chia seeds in four to eight ounces of water twice a day.

An excellent fiber supplement is PGX Fiber. PGX is a unique blend of plant fibers containing glucomannan, a soluble and fermentable fiber derived from the root of the konjac plant. With PGX, I recommend that you start with one capsule three times a day, before meals, with sixteen ounces of water, and gradually increase the dose as tolerated every two to three days. Most people use two to three softgels before meals with sixteen ounces of water. Rarely will someone need six softgels before meals, which is the maximum dose.

Fantastic Fiber

To lower your cholesterol levels, add at least 7 g of fiber to your diet per day. However, start out at a much lower dosage—usually half or a quarter of that amount—to minimize gas or bloating. As your body becomes accustomed to the fiber, gradually increase your intake.

Antioxidant and fatty acid supplements

When LDL cholesterol becomes oxidized, it is much more likely to form plaque on arterial walls. In fact, a new blood test now measures the oxidezed cholesterol, which is most prone to form plaque in the arteries. For this reason, supplementation with antioxidants is extremely important to decrease any damage caused by oxidized LDL cholesterol.

Antioxidants work best when taken together as a team rather than as a single antioxidant. Several antioxidants play an extremely important role in preventing the oxidation of LDL cholesterol. One of the most important is vitamin E in its natural form (d-alpha-tocopherol), which prevents and even reverses the oxidized state of cholesterol. The other seven forms of vitamin E that we discussed before are important as well. Other important antioxidants include alpha lipoic acid, vitamin C, CoQ_{10}, grape seed and pine bark extract, and a glutathione booster, such as N-acetyl cysteine or RiboCeine.

In addition, I also recommend that you take a comprehensive multivitamin.

Niacin

Niacin not only lowers total cholesterol levels, including LDL cholesterol, but it also lowers triglyceride levels and raises high-density lipoprotein (HDL) cholesterol levels. The dose of niacin required to lower cholesterol levels is usually 1,000–3,000 mg a day, and it is best to take a sustained-release niacin supplement, such as Niaspan, or a time-released niacin at a dose of 1,000–3,000 mg at bedtime or after the evening meal. Note: take one to three baby aspirin at the beginning of the meal to prevent flushing.

Unfortunately, because niacin may cause numerous side effects, such as flushing of the skin, ulcers, stomach irritation, elevated liver enzymes, and fatigue, many people are unable to tolerate it. For these individuals, there is another form of niacin called *inositol hexaniacinate*. This form of niacin carries many of the benefits of regular niacin without the side effects.

Inositol hexaniacinate has been used in Europe to lower cholesterol levels and improve blood flow in patients with intermittent calf pain due to poor circulation. Approximately 1,000–1,500 mg per day of inositol hexaniacinate in divided doses is usually adequate for lowering LDL cholesterol and raising HDL cholesterol levels. However, some may need a higher dose. Be sure to consult your physician first before deciding to add any natural "medications" to your lifestyle. If you are taking medication for diabetes, monitor your blood sugar levels closely when taking any form of niacin, even inositol hexaniacinate.

Phytosterols

Phytosterols (plant sterols) effectively interfere with small intestine absorption of cholesterol and therefore, when eaten, can lower a person's LDL cholesterol levels. Seeds, nuts, vegetables, fruits, beans, and legumes all contain adequate amounts of phytosterols that can lower your levels of LDL cholesterol. Phytosterols also are found in many products, including some margarine spreads; all vegetables and vegetable-based products contain phytosterols. Two of the newer margarine products, Benecol and Take Control, are said to lower cholesterol levels by interfering with the absorption of cholesterol from the food that is eaten with the products. Even still, Dr. Joseph Mercola has this to say about Take Control margarine: "Never forget, margarine is liquid plastic. Your brain is 50 percent fat. Do you want liquid plastic incorporated into your brain?"[77]

In their natural state, all phytosterols are bound to the fibers of the plant from which they come. And there is a better way to incorporate these phytosterols into your diet than eating a tub of margarine! As frequently as possible, try to eat foods with phytosterols as they are grown in nature, before they have been processed and refined. I recommend Cardio-Edge, which contains phytosterols, usually two with each meal. This can be found online.

Pantethine

Pantethine is the active, stable form of pantothenic acid, otherwise known as vitamin B_5. It can be used to lower LDL cholesterol and triglyceride levels while increasing HDL levels. It is believed that pantethine inhibits the production of cholesterol and accelerates the breakdown of fatty acids in the body. Pantethine works best when taken at a dose of 300 mg three times a day.

Red yeast rice

Red yeast is a form of yeast that is cultivated on rice, and it contains substances very similar to the active ingredients in statin drugs, the most commonly prescribed medications for elevated cholesterol levels. Clinical trials performed on red yeast rice products showed that they were able to lower total cholesterol levels by an average of 16 percent.

If you choose to use red yeast rice to lower your cholesterol, be sure to obtain it from a reputable nutritional supplement company, and do so *only* under the care of your physician. Be sure to have your liver checked regularly since red yeast rice can elevate liver enzymes. Also, take 100–200 mg of coenzyme Q_{10} (CoQ_{10}) a day when you are taking red yeast rice.

Help for high triglycerides

Fish oils, or omega-3 fats from fish, can lower triglyceride levels by as much as 30 percent.[78] In fact, fish oil is one of the most effective treatments for lowering triglyceride levels and is much safer than medical drug therapy. Fish oil contains eicosapentaenoic acid (EPA) and docosahexaenoic acid (DHA) and is more beneficial than vegetable omega-3 oils such as flaxseed oil. Salmon, mackerel, sardines, and herring contain more omega-3 fats than other fish, but "farm-raised" fish contain very little omega-3 oil because many farms feed their fish soybean meal.

I recommend eating three to four meals of seafood each week, consisting of the fish that are low in mercury. (See sidebar for a list of low-mercury fish.) But do not fry or deep-fry the fish, because that will counteract any of the benefits of the omega-3 fats.

Fish oil also may be obtained in supplement form. To lower your triglycerides, you should take approximately 4,000–5,000 mg per day of fish oil containing both EPA and DHA with the EPA being a higher percentage than DHA.

Low-Mercury Fish

Choose from this list of fish low in mercury:

Salmon	Tilapia	Shrimp
Catfish	Pollock	Cod[79]

Remember that many fish oil supplements sold over the counter are rancid, meaning that you will not get the beneficial effects from them that you need. A simple test to tell if a fish oil capsule is rancid is to stick a needle into it and then smell it. If it has a very fishy odor, it is rancid. Also, fish oil capsules should contain d-alpha-tocopherol (a natural vitamin E) in the ingredient list and may also contain rosemary extract to prevent rancidity. Soluble fiber also helps lower triglyceride levels.

HYPERTENSION (HIGH BLOOD PRESSURE)

Supplements are an essential part of the battle against hypertension, more commonly known as high blood pressure. Free-radical damage contributes to hypertension and atherosclerosis. Taking supplements can greatly strengthen your body's ability to battle the devastating effects of free radicals.

When high blood pressure goes untreated for too long, your arteries eventually lose their elasticity and actually begin to form plaque. The hypertension causes shearing forces that injure the lining of the arterial walls, causing the buildup of even more plaque. More and more plaque builds up until arteries eventually become blocked or the plaque ruptures, forming a blood clot, triggering a heart attack or stroke.

This is why controlling hypertension is so important. Having a proper diet is important in controlling hypertension. (Please refer to my books *The New Bible Cure for Hypertension* and *Let Your Food Be Your Medicine*, and follow the anti-inflammatory Mediterranean diet for hypertension.) On top of your diet, antioxidants and supplements are critically important in controlling blood pressure usually without any side effects. Let's look at some of these powerful defenders.

Coenzyme Q_{10}

Coenzyme Q_{10} (CoQ_{10}) has several benefits for the cardiovascular system that help lower blood pressure and normalize heart contraction and rhythm. It also helps improve energy production at the cellular level by improving mitochondrial function. The mitochondria are like tiny energy factories inside each cell. Heart muscle cells have the most mitochondria because they never stop working. Individuals with hypertension, or high blood pressure, are often deficient in CoQ_{10}.

Research has shown that CoQ_{10} reduces blood pressure. In one study subjects experienced significantly improved systolic and diastolic pressure and an overall improvement of heart function. Some were able to completely stop their blood pressure medication four months after starting supplementation with CoQ_{10}.

As we age, CoQ_{10} levels decline, so older people should always be checked out to determine potential CoQ_{10} deficiency. I commonly check CoQ_{10} blood levels on elderly patients with heart disease. Certain medications used for cardiovascular conditions actually deplete the body of CoQ_{10}: thiazide diuretics, beta-blockers, clonidine, methyldopa, and especially cholesterol-lowering agents such as statin medications (statin) and fenofibrates.

I recommend the active form of CoQ_{10} (ubiquinol), 100 to 200 mg one or two times a day.

L-arginine

L-arginine is an amino acid that improves blood flow and improves the activity of the endothelial cells. The endothelium is the layer of cells that line the interior surface of blood vessels and is very thin, only one cell thick, and very fragile. When the endothelium is well nourished, optimal amounts of nitric oxide (NO) are produced by these endothelial cells. NO helps maintain the elasticity of all blood vessels and especially the arteries. NO is also a signaling molecule that signals arteries to dilate, which helps lower blood pressure. L-arginine is converted to NO in the body; however, one cannot consume adequate amounts of L-arginine from food alone. Arginine is present in red meat, chicken, fish, soy nuts, beans, and dairy.

The typical dose of L-arginine to lower blood pressure is 2–3 g or more twice a day, in the morning and at bedtime, on an empty stomach.

L-citrulline

This is another amino acid that is very similar to L-arginine and is also present in red meats, chicken, and fish, but it is also present in melons, especially watermelon, and highest in watermelon seed. L-citrulline is converted in the body to L-arginine, which increases the production of NO. When L-arginine is combined with L-citrulline, NO output is actually increased significantly. There is an L-citrulline/L-arginine recycling pathway that boosts NO production beyond when taking either L-arginine or L-citrulline alone. This is the reason I recommend that these two amino acids be taken together. The typical dose of L-citrulline to lower blood pressure is 200–1,000 mg or approximately 500 mg once or twice a day, but remember, it works much better if combined with L-arginine and taken on an empty stomach.

Olive leaf extract

The active ingredient in olive leaf is oleuropein, which functions as an ACE inhibitor, which is a major group of blood pressure medicines. Oleuropein has been shown to modulate the core cause of high blood pressure: arterial resistance or stiffness. One study showed that people with hypertension could experience reduced systolic blood pressure by an average of 11.5 points mmHg, and diastolic blood pressure by 4.8 points—in just eight weeks—by taking olive leaf extract in a dose of 500 mg twice a day.[80]

Beetroot powder

Drinking just one teaspoon of beetroot powder in 4 ounces of water can help lower your blood pressure by boosting nitric oxide levels. Beetroot naturally contains high levels of nitrate, and nitrate has an enormous effect on lowering blood pressure. Nitrate increases the levels of nitric oxide in the bloodstream. Nitric oxide relaxes and widens the blood vessels, therefore improving blood pressure.[81] In a study in the journal *Hypertension* in February 2015 sixty-four hypertensive patients drank an eight-ounce glass of beetroot juice every morning for one month. The average drop in systolic blood pressure was 8 mmHg, which is significant. One teaspoon of beetroot powder is usually equivalent to three beets. I recommend one teaspoon of beetroot powder twice a day in four ounces of water. It is my favorite supplement for lowering blood pressure.

Hibiscus

According to a study discussed in *Phytomedicine,* consuming tea made from the extract of hibiscus may lower a person's blood pressure. This tea needs to be consumed every day. It lowers blood pressure because it is a diuretic and a mild blood vessel dilator.

In this study seventy individuals with hypertension were chosen at random to consume either hibiscus tea or captopril, an antihypertensive medication, for four weeks. After the four weeks tests confirmed these two treatments are similar in their effectiveness—the medication reduced the blood pressure in 84 percent of individuals, and the hibiscus tea did the same in 79 percent of individuals.

These results combined with the safety and low chance of experiencing side effects shows that hibiscus tea is an effective treatment and may be an alternative to medication for some individuals.[82]

Celery seed extract

Celery seed extract has powerful calcium-channel blocking properties, which is a major group of blood pressure medicines. Celery seed extract has been shown in clinical studies to lower blood pressure. A compound in celery seed L-3-n-butylphthalide (3nB) is the key compound to lower blood pressure. In one study thirty hypertensive men took 75 mg of celery seed extract twice daily for six weeks. That is the equivalent of 530 stalks of celery. After three weeks the blood pressure dropped an average of 8.2 mmHg systolic and 8.5 mmHg diastolic.[83] Celery seed also appears to improve blood flow to the brain and prevent strokes. I recommend 75 mg of celery seed extract twice a day.

Critical minerals

Sodium

For over twenty years Americans with hypertension have been warned to limit sodium in their diets. Numerous studies have confirmed that a low-sodium diet lowers blood pressure if you are "sodium sensitive."[84]

Sodium controls the amount of fluid outside the cells and regulates the body's water balance and blood volume. Your kidneys actually regulate the amount of sodium in your body. When your sodium level is low, your kidneys begin to conserve sodium. When levels become high, your kidneys excrete the excess sodium in the urine.

Salt is the most common source of sodium. It is made up of approximately 60 percent chloride and 40 percent sodium. Your body requires about 500 mg of sodium every day, which is approximately a quarter of a teaspoon of salt a day. But Americans consume between 3,000 and 4,000 mg a day and on average 3,400 mg a day.

A simplified analogy to understand blood pressure is to simply envision a garden hose with a nozzle on it. There are only two ways to increase the pressure in the hose. You can either turn the faucet so that maximum water flows out of the faucet, or you can tighten the nozzle on the end of the hose. Your blood pressure usually rises the same way. If you consume too much salt or high-sodium foods, you typically retain more water, and the blood pressure rises similar to when you opened the faucet up and increased the flow of water through the hose. The increased volume of blood then forces the heart to work harder, leading to increased resistance in the arteries, which, in turn, leads to high blood pressure. Limiting sodium intake to 2,300 mg or less a day, or for some 1,500 mg a day, will lower one's blood pressure 11.4/5.7 mmHg—that is pretty significant. It lowers blood pressure as much as most blood pressure medications but without any side effects!

Potassium

Potassium is another mineral that helps lower blood pressure. It also helps keep your body's sodium level down to acceptable levels. That's why eating foods high in potassium, such as fresh fruits and vegetables, can help protect against high blood pressure. Foods such as tomatoes, avocados, and beans (especially lima beans and organic soybeans) are high in potassium. Also, a form of seaweed called dulse is extremely high in potassium. More than 4,000 mg of potassium is found in one-sixth of a cup! You can find dulse at your favorite health food store.

Magnesium

Magnesium is vital for healthy blood pressure and a robust cardiovascular system. This powerful mineral is linked to more than 325 different enzyme reactions in the body. If your body is deficient in magnesium, you could be predisposed to developing hypertension, arrhythmias, and other cardiovascular conditions. Magnificent magnesium actually dilates arteries, thus decreasing blood pressure.

For this reason, I strongly recommend taking a magnesium supplement. Take 200 mg of a chelated form, such as magnesium glycinate, magnesium citrate, or magnesium aspartate, once or twice a day. Let me caution you, however, that too much magnesium may cause diarrhea.

Common sources of magnesium include nuts and seeds, green leafy vegetables, legumes, and whole grains.

Calcium

Did you know that the most abundant mineral in your body is calcium? Calcium is critically important for maintaining the balance between your sodium and potassium and for regulating your blood pressure.

You can increase the amount of calcium in your diet by eating calcium-rich foods, such as almonds, skim milk, and more. Or, try taking a daily calcium magnesium supplement containing 200 mg of calcium and 100 mg of magnesium two to three times a day. New studies are finding that consuming too much calcium in foods and supplements can increase the risk of heart attack and stroke. So don't overdo it on calcium supplements, and don't consume excessive dairy products.

Water

Believe it or not, one of the best nutrients you can take for lowering or controlling your blood pressure is water.

When your body is lacking water, the water volume in every cell will be reduced, which then affects how efficiently nutrients and waste products are transported. What happens in the end is that our cells don't get enough nutrients, and they end up having too much waste collecting in them.

In addition, when you don't have enough water, your kidneys reabsorb more sodium. After you do drink fluids, this sodium, in turn, attracts and holds even more water, making the blood volume increase, which, in turn, may increase your blood pressure. It is similar to turning up the faucet to increase the flow of water.

If you don't drink enough water for too long, your body will begin to make certain adjustments to keep adequate blood flowing to your brain, heart, kidneys, liver, and lungs. Blood will be shunted away from less essential tissues and sent to the vital organs. Your body will actually divert water by constricting small arteries that lead to less essential tissues. In other words, your body will begin a water-rationing program to make sure that enough blood goes to the vital organs first.

Think of it like this: when you constrict a water hose by bending it or by pressing your thumb over the opening, what happens? The pressure behind that constriction increases dramatically, doesn't it? Your arteries behave in a similar way. Therefore, increasing your intake of water helps open up your smaller arteries and helps prevent this rise in blood pressure.

Often an individual with mild hypertension is placed on medication when all he really needs is to drink more water. When high blood pressure is detected early enough, simply drinking two to three quarts of alkaline or spring water a day usually can bring it back to normal. Avoid distilled or reverse osmosis water if you have hypertension since they are very acidic and usually void of minerals.

What's even worse than medicating a person who just needs water is placing such an individual on diuretics, which happens all the time. They lose even more water as well as valuable electrolytes, including potassium and magnesium.

If you have high blood pressure, drink at least eight to twelve glasses of alkaline or spring water a day. The best time to drink water is thirty minutes before meals and two hours after meals. However, if you have kidney disease or a weak heart, you will need to limit your water intake, and you should be under the care of a physician.

IRRITABLE BOWEL SYNDROME (IBS)

Most of our lives are too full of cares, hurts, obstacles, disappointments, and other stressors. All of these emotions can release themselves right into our gut, resulting in IBS that becomes increasingly chronic. To begin the healing process and physical renewal, you must target one of the places where stress can create the most havoc—your gastrointestinal (GI) tract. You can do this with the help of powerful supplements that will go right to work to soothe and heal the damage. Most patients with IBS also suffer from food sensitivities, especially gluten, and should have an ALCAT to identify their food sensitivities. Also many patients with IBS have candida overgrowth or small intestinal bacterial overgrowth or parasites.

Let's look at some supplements that are vital for your recovery.

Good bacteria

When you suffer with IBS, supplementing your body's own good bacteria is essential. It may be hard to believe that more than four hundred different kinds of bacteria are living in your colon right now. These friendly bacteria are necessary to health.

The most important friendly bacteria are the lactobacillus acidophilus and bifidobacterium. To increase their presence in your digestive tract, you can take them as supplements. I recommend L-acidophilus and bifidobacterium as well as other strains of probiotics. See appendix A. I usually recommend at least 50–100 billion colony-forming units a day or more on an empty stomach upon awakening.

Prebiotics

Prebiotics feed the probiotics, or good bacteria. Fructooligosaccharides (FOS), a type of prebiotic, are sugars that promote the growth of good bacteria. They are found in plants such as banana, garlic, and more.[85] I usually recommend about 2,000 mg of FOS daily taken with the probiotic. This supplement can be found in most health food stores. Inulin and chicory are also good prebiotics. Chia seed is also an excellent prebiotic, and I recommend one tablespoon two times a day, again taken with the probiotic.

Slippery elm

Slippery elm is an herb used to soothe irritated tissues, such as inflammation in the small or large bowel. Slippery elm can be consumed as tea or taken in its herbal form in a veggie capsule. Just avoid gelatin capsules since these can aggravate IBS. You may take slippery elm lozenges three times per day.

Glutamine

When treating IBS, it's extremely important to repair the lining of the small intestine or heal the leaky gut. The amino acid glutamine is one of the most important supplements for repairing the GI tract.

I usually recommend 500–1,000 mg thirty minutes before meals two or three times a day. Take a veggie capsule or powder form.

Supplements for depression and anxiety

Excess stress, anxiety, or depression also may be associated with IBS. Let's look at some supplements that can help. If you are battling depression, select one supplement from the following list:

- 5-HTP (50 mg three times per day) or 150 mg at bedtime
- SAM-e (200–800 mg two times per day on an empty stomach)
- St. John's wort (300 mg three times per day)

Don't take any of these supplements if you are taking a prescription antidepressant medicine. Please refer to my booklet *The Bible Cure for Depression and Anxiety.*

An excellent supplement for anxiety and stress is Stress Relief Drops. This supplement is not addictive like medications such as Xanax and Valium. It does not impair mental functioning, and it works well for anxiety and stress. Take ten drops in two ounces of water as needed. See appendix A.

Overcoming constipation

IBS sufferers tend to spend much of their time dealing with either constipation or diarrhea or both at different times. Dealing with constipation in a natural, healthy way will help.

Many people are dependent upon laxatives to have a bowel movement. If you are among them, it is essential to restore your body to normal functioning. Avoid all stimulant laxatives, including herbal laxatives such as senna and cascara sagrada. These remedies stimulate the bowel muscles to contract, which may actually worsen symptoms of IBS.

The safest laxatives are the bulk-forming varieties of various kinds of fiber.

Fiber

Most fibers that I use for IBS patients contain a combination of both soluble and insoluble fiber. Insoluble fiber improves the transit time of the GI tract and helps to sweep the colon clean. Avoid all fibers that contain wheat since gluten sensitivity is very common in most of the patients that I see with IBS. The insoluble fiber also helps remove yeast, bad bacteria, and parasites, literally sweeping them out of the colon. Soluble fiber, on the other hand, binds toxins, including bacterial and yeast toxins and carcinogens in our food, and prevents them from being reabsorbed by our GI tract.

1. *Rice bran.* This is a wonderful source of fiber for those with a sensitive GI tract. I recommend starting with one tablespoon of rice bran a day, gradually increasing the dosage to two tablespoons two times per day.
2. *The husks of psyllium seeds.* You can find this fiber source in many over-the-counter preparations. They are an excellent source of both insoluble and soluble fiber. (Avoid brands that contain sugar or NutraSweet.) Start introducing this fiber into your diet slowly by taking only one teaspoon a day. Gradually increase the amount to one tablespoon two times a day.
3. *Chia seeds or ground flaxseed.* Taking one tablespoon of chia seeds or ground flaxseed one to three times per day is excellent for constipation. I prefer chia seeds since they do not have to be ground up.

Supplements will go right to work supporting, relaxing, and soothing your GI tract. However, gelatin capsules and caplets may aggravate IBS in some patients; if so, they should be avoided. Many patients with IBS have candida and food sensitivities. Please refer to *The Bible Cure for Candida and Yeast Infections* and the antigen leukocyte cellular antibody test (ALCAT) to identify food sensitivities. Please refer to the FODMAP diet in appendix B for the best diet for IBS.

Memory Loss

Age-related memory loss often starts at about forty-five to fifty years of age. Nearly 15 percent of people experiencing progressive age-related memory loss go on to develop Alzheimer's disease. While some treat memory loss as an inevitable part of aging, that isn't true. Good nutrition, healthy lifestyle choices, exercise, vitamins, and supplements can empower you to halt the debilitating effects of memory loss. I take all patients with memory loss off gluten, MSG, and NutraSweet, and have them follow the diet in *Let Food Be Your Medicine*.

Taking the right supplements is especially vital to arresting and reversing the situation. This is particularly true for antioxidants, which fight free radicals. The brain generates more free radicals than any other tissue in the body. Dr. Lester Packer, who served as head of the Packer Lab, professor and senior researcher at University of California at Berkeley for forty years, believes that the body's best defense against free radicals is a network of antioxidants. Dr.

Packer sees five extraordinary ones as making up this network. They include vitamin E, lipoic acid, vitamin C, glutathione, and coenzyme Q_{10} (CoQ_{10}).[86]

These five join together to form an impenetrable shield against free-radical attacks. When one antioxidant fails to neutralize a free-radical hit, another launches to back it up. Vitamin C or CoQ_{10} can donate electrons to revive a failed vitamin E hit. And lipoic acid can resuscitate all the other antioxidants in addition to itself.

The defense team

The brain-protecting antioxidant defense team can be taken as daily supplements. If you've been experiencing some symptoms of memory loss, beginning this supplementation regimen may give you immediate relief. Let's take a closer look.

Vitamin E

Vitamin E protects the fat in cell membranes from turning rancid. In April 1997 the *New England Journal of Medicine* reported that the debilitating symptoms of Alzheimer's disease were reduced in half of Alzheimer's patients who took 1,000 IU of vitamin E daily.[87]

Some experts say that about 30 percent of Americans have a vitamin E deficiency. In addition, all developed countries are slightly deficient in vitamin E.[88] Take 400 IU of natural vitamin E with all eight forms of vitamin E daily for antioxidant protection. Dosages of 800 IU or more may thin the blood. Therefore, check with your physician before taking more than 400 IU.

Vitamin C

The antioxidant vitamin C actually donates electrons to help regenerate vitamin E. The brain also uses vitamin C to make the neurotransmitters dopamine and adrenaline. Vitamin C also increases levels of glutathione, which is one of the most important antioxidants in the body.

Take 500 mg of vitamin C two to three times a day.

Coenzyme Q_{10} (CoQ_{10})

CoQ_{10} is an extremely important brain-enhancing antioxidant because it protects the fats in the brain from turning rancid. This free-radical damage, called lipid peroxidation, can kill brain cells. CoQ_{10} also helps recycle vitamin E, and it helps produce energy in the brain. CoQ_{10} quenches free radicals before they damage nerve cell membranes.

Take at least 100–200 mg of CoQ_{10} a day. If you smoke, if you're experiencing memory loss, or if you have heart disease, take at least 200–400 mg or more of CoQ_{10} daily.

Alpha lipoic acid

Lipoic acid is one of the most powerful antioxidants. It easily penetrates the blood-brain barrier in the fatty and water-soluble portions of cells. It is also the only antioxidant that can recycle itself.

Lipoic acid not only neutralizes free radicals, but it also increases the efficiency of mitochondria. This powerful defender helps control insulin and blood sugar by preventing advanced glycation end products (AGEs), which we know tend to accelerate aging and memory loss.

Take at least 600 mg of alpha lipoic acid daily, 300 mg in the morning and 300 mg in the afternoon. If you are diabetic, you may increase that dosage to 600 mg three times a day. Be sure and monitor thyroid tests if you take the higher dose of lipoic acid.

Glutathione

The fifth powerful antioxidant the brain needs daily is glutathione. But it's not easy to increase levels of this powerful antioxidant with food or supplements. Taking lipoic acid will actually raise your glutathione levels, and it will help your body recycle the glutathione that it already has.

Glutathione supplements are poorly absorbed, and I do not recommend them. Supplements of N-acetyl cysteine can raise your glutathione, and I recommend 500–1,000 mg twice a day. However, RiboCeine is the best glutathione booster. (See appendix A.)

Acetyl L-carnitine

Carnitine is a vitamin-like substance that's used for conditions such as congestive heart failure and angina. Acetyl L-carnitine (ALC) is a special form of carnitine that aids mental functioning.

ALC increases energy across the brain's mitochondrial membrane, and it improves communication between the brain's two hemispheres. ALC appears to be much more effective for patients with early age-associated memory impairment.

If you are experiencing mild memory impairment, take 500 mg of ALC two or three times a day. If you are experiencing moderate to severe memory impairment, take 500–1,000 mg two or three times a day.

Phosphatidylserine (PS)

Phosphatidylserine (PS) is a phospholipid that plays an important role in cell membrane function. It enables brain cells to metabolize glucose and release neurotransmitters. It is essential to the brain's ability to send and receive chemical communication. But as we age, production of PS decreases, and one eventually can become deficient in PS. Two large clinical studies concluded that PS could provide significant benefits for cognitive functions that usually decline with age, including memory, learning, concentration, and vocabulary skills. Supplementation with 100 mg of PS three times a day has been shown to improve cognitive performance in patients with age-associated memory impairment.[89]

Curcumin

Curcumin is the pigment that gives the brilliant yellow color to the spice turmeric. It is one of the most powerful anti-inflammatory compounds in nature. In a study of over one thousand residents over the age of sixty in Singapore, the residents had not been diagnosed with any form of dementia; they took a diet survey and then were evaluated using the Mini Mental State Examination for Alzheimer's. Those who often consumed curry had a 49 percent lower risk of cognitive problems compared with those who never or rarely ate curry.[90]

The rate of Alzheimer's disease in the Indian population is among the lowest in the world and only a fourth of the rate in the United States. I strongly believe it is because curry is commonly consumed by the people of India. James A. Duke, PhD, published a comprehensive summary of over seven hundred turmeric studies. Turmeric (curcumin) was found to counteract symptoms of Alzheimer's disease by blocking the formation of beta-amyloid, the sticky protein associated with Alzheimer's disease.[91] I usually recommend 250–1,000 mg of curcumin two times a day or sometimes three times a day.

Pyrroloquinoline quinone (PQQ)

PQQ is the next-generation coenzyme and is one of the most exciting supplements discovered because it not only protects the mitochondria (the energy factories in every cell) from oxidative damage (free radicals) but also stimulates the growth of new mitochondria, even in aging cells. PQQ also protects the brain and optimizes the health and function of the entire central nervous system. PQQ was able to reverse cognitive impairment caused by chronic oxidative stress. PQQ also protects the brain from neurotoxins, including mercury. PQQ stimulates the production and release of nerve growth factor in cells that support neurons in the brain. It has also been shown to protect memory and cognition in aging humans and animals.[92] I recommend 20 mg of PQQ once or twice a day.

Menopause

For the majority of women, menopause occurs at about fifty years of age. However, it can occur as early as thirty-five or forty, and may occur as late as fifty-five or sixty. If you are going through menopause, or are in perimenopause, you may be experiencing mood swings, along with such bothersome symptoms as hot flashes, night sweats, fatigue, headaches, or heart palpitations. I strongly recommend that you start bioidentical hormone replacement therapy (BHRT). To find a a medical doctor trained in BHRT, go to worldhealth.net or see appendix A.

Vitamins and supplements for menopause

Taking certain vitamins and supplements will greatly reduce any of the adverse symptoms of menopause. The following list of vitamins and supplements usually will help relieve menopausal symptoms.

Vitamin E

Taken internally at a dosage of 800 IU daily, vitamin E may help menopausal symptoms. Vitamin E cream applied to the vaginal area may prevent itching.

Vitamin C

Vitamin C with bioflavonoids, such as hesperidin and quercetin, may help relieve hot flashes. Take at least 1,000 mg daily of both vitamin C and bioflavonoids in divided doses.

Evening primrose oil, borage oil, and black currant seed oil

These oils also may relieve hot flashes. You should take enough evening primrose, borage, or black currant oil to equal 300 mg of the fatty gamma-linolenic acid (GLA) a day.

A multivitamin/multimineral supplement

I recommend this for menopausal women.

Calcium

I used to recommend calcium in a dose of 1,500 mg a day with at least 400 units to 5,000 IU of vitamin D. I now recommend 200–250 mg of calcium three times a day and vitamin K_2 100 mg a day to regulate calcium metabolism.

Bioidentical progesterone

This can be taken either in cream form from a health food store or prescribed by a physician. Make sure it is bioidentical, however. Use at least 30 mg of bioidentical progesterone cream once or twice a day. Progesterone helps boost estrogen levels mildly, helping to relieve hot flashes. I usually recommend 3 to 6 percent progesterone cream. Do not use synthetic progesterone.

Herbs that can help

Herbs also may be helpful in controlling menopausal symptoms.

Black cohosh

This comes from a shrub that is native to the forests of North America. Its black root is one of the main constituents used in the herbal preparation. The word *cohosh* is an Indian word that means "rough." Native American

Indians used this herb for many different problems, including menopausal symptoms, menstrual cramps, and even rattlesnake bites.

During menopause, estrogen production usually slows down and another hormone, called LH, or the luteinizing hormone, increases. As a result of the increasing LH and decreasing estrogen, hot flashes occur.

Black cohosh has weak estrogen-like activity, and it may decrease the LH secretion, thus reducing hot flashes. I recommend the standardized extract of the herb, which contains 1 mg per tablet.

An excellent product that contains black cohosh is Remifemin. It is found in most health food stores.

Dong quai

This is a plant that is a member of the celery family. It is often referred to in Chinese medicine as female ginseng. It tends to help balance the feminine hormonal system. Dong quai is not a phytoestrogen like soy and does not exhibit any hormone-like actions in the body. Dong quai helps relieve hot flashes during the perimenopausal period. By balancing female hormones, it usually helps to relieve painful menstruation or too frequent menstruation.

The root of the plant is used for medicinal purposes. The powdered root can be purchased at a health food store in capsule, tablet, or tea forms. A common dose of dong quai capsules is 1–2 g three times a day.

Chasteberry

Also called vitex, chasteberry has been used since ancient times to suppress libido and inspire chastity. The whole-fruit extract of the chasteberry is used. The chasteberry contains no hormones. However, it is believed to be able to increase production of progesterone, thus helping to regulate a woman's menstrual cycle.

Chasteberry does not work rapidly. It usually takes months for this berry to start balancing the woman's hormonal system. Powdered extracts are usually taken in a dose of 250–500 mg three times a day.

Estrovera

Estrovera is a nonhormonal supplement for women dealing with menopause that has been used in Europe for over twenty years. It contains an extract from rhubarb and has been shown to help with symptoms of menopause.[93] Rhubarb has been shown to help reduce the number and intensity of hot flashes.[94] The dose is one capsule a day.

Flaxseed

Take two to three tablespoons of ground flaxseed one to three times a day. This helps by boosting phytoestrogens, which exert an effect similar to that of estrogen. Flaxseed has been shown to help with hot flashes as well as other symptoms of menopause.[95] My favorite three supplements for menopausal syptoms are black cohosh, Estrovera, and flaxseed.

Bioidentical hormone replacement

If the above natural supplements and herbs are not relieving your hot flashes, I recommend bioidentical hormone replacement by an anti-aging physician. These include bioidentical estrogen, bioidentical progesterone, and bioidentical testosterone. To find a doctor trained in bioidentical hormone replacement, go to worldhealth.net and find a board-certified physician in anti-aging medicine.

OBESITY/OVERWEIGHT

Even though I addressed metabolism and weight in chapter 5, it is worth addressing obesity and ways of dealing with overweight conditions through supplements. Since there are many causes of obesity, I recommend safe nutritional supplements that work through different mechanisms, such as thermogenic agents, natural appetite suppressants that increase satiety, supplements that increase insulin sensitivity, and energy products.

A good multivitamin and multimineral

It's important to be sure that you get a good supply of all the various vitamins your body needs, especially if it is depleted. Most multivitamins contain only twelve vitamins in their inactive form. You may want to choose a multivitamin you can take two to three times a day. To prevent our adrenal glands from becoming exhausted, we need to supplement our diets daily with a comprehensive multivitamin and mineral formula with adequate amounts of B-complex vitamins.

Thermogenic (fat-burning) agents

The term *thermogenic* describes the body's natural means of raising its temperature to burn off more calories. More specifically, thermogenesis is the process of triggering the body to burn white body fat, which is the kind of fat we often accumulate as we age. Thermogenic agents, then, are fat burners that help increase the rate of white-body-fat breakdown. Fortunately most unsafe thermogenic agents have been pulled off the market.

Green tea

Green tea and green tea extract are good weight-loss supplements. Green tea has been used for thousands of years in Asia as both a tea and an herbal medicine. It has two key ingredients: a catechin called epigallocatechin gallate (EGCG) and caffeine. Both lead to the release of more epinephrine, which then increases the metabolic rate. Ultimately green tea promotes fat oxidation, which is fat burning. It also increases the rate at which you burn calories over a twenty-four-hour period.

An effective daily dose of EGCG is 90 mg or more, which can be consumed by drinking three or four cups of green tea a day. Do not add sugar, honey, or artificial sweeteners to it, though you may use the natural sweetener stevia. In addition to drinking green tea, I recommend 100 mg of green tea supplement three times a day.

Green coffee bean extract

A placebo-controlled study reported in January 2012 that green coffee bean extract produced weight loss in 100 percent of overweight participants. For twenty-two weeks, participants were given 350 mg of green coffee bean extract twice a day. They did not change their diets, averaging 2,400 calories per day, but they did burn 400 calories a day through exercise. The average weight loss was 17.6 pounds, with some subjects losing 22.7 pounds, and there were no side effects.[96]

The key phytonutrient in green coffee bean extract is chlorogenic acid, which has the ability to decrease the uptake of glucose, fats, and carbohydrates from the intestines and thus decrease the absorption of calories. It also has positive effects on how your body processes glucose and fats, and it helps lower blood sugar and insulin levels. Drinking coffee doesn't give you the same effects. Because of roasting, most of the chlorogenic acid in coffee is destroyed. By comparison, the extract is much better. Green coffee bean extract should contain 45 percent or more of chlorogenic acid. In addition to—or in place of—drinking coffee, I recommend taking 400 mg of green coffee bean extract thirty minutes before each meal.

Thyroid support

All obese patients should be screened for hypothyroidism, using tests such as the blood tests thyroid-stimulating hormone (TSH), free T3, free T4, Reverse T3, and thyroid peroxidase antibodies to rule out Hashimoto's thyroiditis, the most common cause of low thyroid. If a patient has low body temperature (less than 98 degrees), he or she most likely has a sluggish metabolism and may have sluggish thyroid function.

It's especially important to optimize the free T3 blood level to improve the metabolic rate. The normal range of T3, according to the lab I use, is 2.1–4.4. I try to optimize the T3 level to a range of 3.0–4.2 by using both T4 and natural thyroid extract (T3). I can sometimes optimize the T3 levels with natural supplements, including Metabolic Advantage or iodine supplements, such as Lugol's Iodine. I also commonly perform a lab test to see if a patient is low in iodine before starting iodine supplements. According to the American Thyroid Association, 40 percent of the world's population is at risk for iodine deficiency.[97]

Appetite suppressants

These supplements generally act on the central nervous system to decrease appetite or create a sensation of fullness. Although some medications in this category include risk-prone phenylpropanolamine (found in such products as Dexatrim), I have found a few safe, natural supplements that are extremely effective appetite suppressants.

L-tryptophan and 5-HTP

These are amino acids that help the body to manufacture serotonin. Serotonin assists in controlling carbohydrate and sugar cravings. L-tryptophan and 5-HTP also function like natural antidepressants. If you are taking migraine medications called triptans or selective serotonin reuptake inhibitors (SSRIs), you should talk with your physician before taking either supplement. The typical dose of L-tryptophan is 500–2,000 mg at bedtime. For 5-HTP, it is typically 50–100 mg one to three times a day or 100–300 mg at bedtime.

L-tyrosine, N-acetyl L-tyrosine, and L-phenylalanine

These are naturally occurring amino acids found in numerous protein foods, including cottage cheese, turkey, and chicken. They help raise norepinephrine and dopamine levels in the brain, which then helps decrease appetite and cravings and improves your mood. Doses of L-tyrosine, N-acetyl L-tyrosine, and L-phenylalanine may range from 500–2,000 mg a day (sometimes higher), but they should be taken on an empty stomach. I prefer N-acetyl L-tyrosine for most of my patients since the body absorbs it better than L-tyrosine or L-phenylalanine.

I typically start patients on 500–1,000 mg of N-acetyl L-tyrosine, taken thirty minutes before breakfast and thirty minutes before lunch. I do not recommend taking any of these supplements in late afternoon because they may interfere with sleep.

Mucuna

While traditionally used to treat depression or Parkinson's disease, this supplement also may be of some use to help people lose weight. It has been shown to increase dopamine levels.[98] Low dopamine is associated with craving sugar, chocolate, and carbohydrates.[99] Raising dopamine with mucuna will help eliminate food cravings and therefore help people lose weight. I recommend mucuna containing 60 percent L-dopamine in a 100 mg capsule. Simply take the one capsule in the morning, thirty minutes before breakfast. Do not take more than two capsules a day.

Supplements to increase satiety

Fiber supplements and foods high in fiber increase feelings of fullness by using several different mechanisms. Fiber slows the passage of food through the digestive tract, decreases the absorption of sugars and starches into the stomach, and expands and fills up the stomach—turning down the appetite. Although the American Heart Association and the National Cancer Institute recommend 30 g or more of fiber each day, the average American consumes only from 12–17 g.[100]

When it comes to losing weight and managing blood sugar levels, a little fiber goes a long way. One study found that consuming an extra 14 g of soluble fiber each day for only two days was associated with a 10 percent decrease in caloric intake.[101] Soluble-fiber supplements significantly increase post-meal satisfaction and should be taken before each meal to assist in weight loss. Soluble fiber lowers the blood sugar, slowing down digestion and the absorption of sugars and carbohydrates. This allows for a more gradual rise in blood sugar, which lowers the glycemic index of the foods you eat. This helps improve the blood sugar levels.

The fiber that I prefer for weight-loss patients is PolyGlycopleX (PGX). I start with one capsule, taken with eight to sixteen ounces of water before each meal and snack, and then gradually increase the dose to two to four capsules until patients can control their appetite. Always take PGX with evening meals and snacks.

In addition to PGX, another great fiber for weight loss is glucomannan, made from the Asian root konjac. Glucomannan is five times more effective in lowering cholesterol when compared with other fibers such as psyllium, oat fiber, or guar gum. Because it expands to ten times its original size when placed in water, it is a great supplement to take before a meal to reduce your appetite as it expands in your stomach, but you should take it with 16 ounces of water or unsweetened black or green tea. Another great and inexpensive fiber is chia seeds, and I recommend one tablespoon in four to eight ounces of water before or after each meal.

Supplements to increase energy production

L-carnitine is an amino acid that helps our bodies turn food into energy by shuttling fatty acids into the mitochondria, which act as our cells' energy factories by burning fatty acids for energy. Humans synthesize very little carnitine, so we may need to supplement from outside sources. This applies especially to obese and older individuals, who typically have lower levels of carnitine than the average-weight segment of the population. As you might expect, individuals with insufficient carnitine have a greater difficulty burning fat for energy.

Milk, meat such as mutton and lamb, fish, and cheese are good sources of L-carnitine. In supplement form, I recommend taking a combination of L-carnitine and acetyl L-carnitine, and alpha lipoic acid. I recommend 500 mg each L-carnitine and acetyl L-carnitine 300 mg of alpha lipoic acid twice a day. The best time to take these supplements is in the morning and early afternoon (before 3:00 p.m.) on an empty stomach. If you take them any later, these supplements can impair your sleep. Green tea supplements and N-acetyl L-tyrosine also help increase your energy.

Other supplements that boost energy include coenzyme Q_{10} (CoQ10), PQQ, and RiboCeine (glutathione-boosting supplement).

Other weight-loss supplements

There are a couple of other supplements that may help on your weight-loss journey.

Irvingia

Irvingia is a fruit-bearing plant grown in the jungles of Cameroon in Africa. *Irvingia gabonensis* helps resensitize your cells to insulin. It appears to be able to reverse leptin resistance by lowering levels of C-reactive protein (CRP), an inflammatory mediator. Leptin is a hormone that tells your brain you've eaten enough and that it is time to stop. It also enhances your body's ability to use fat as an energy source. One also needs zinc, 12–15 mg a day, which is present in most comprehensive multivitamins, in order for leptin to function optimally.

Because of Americans' sedentary lifestyles and highly processed, high-glycemic food choices, many overweight and obese patients have acquired resistance to leptin. As a result, this hormone no longer works properly in their bodies. Similar to insulin resistance, leptin resistance is a chronic inflammatory condition that contributes to weight gain. It is critically important to follow an anti-inflammatory dietary program (outlined in my book *The New Bible Cure for Weight Loss*). Simply decreasing inflammatory foods enables most to start losing belly fat and also allows leptin to function optimally. The generally recommended dose is 150 mg of standardized *Irvingia* extract twice a day, thirty minutes before lunch and dinner.

7-keto DHEA

Derived from the hormone dehydroepiandrosterone (DHEA), 7-keto DHEA is taken to help rev a person's metabolism to aid in weight loss. Unlike its DHEA, which is produced by glands near the kidneys, 7-keto DHEA does not affect sex hormone levels.[102] The supplement also is used to improve lean body mass, build muscle, boost the immune system, enhance memory, and slow aging, though there is limited scientific evidence to support all of those benefits.[103] However, 7-keto DHEA has been shown to increase the resting metabolic rate in those who were already dieting and engaging in regular exercise.

An eight-week study found that those who took 100 mg of 7-keto DHEA twice a day lost about six pounds, while those who received a placebo lost a little over two pounds.[104] The supplement was not found to have any adverse side effects after a series of toxicological evaluations. A safety study published in *Clinical Investigative Medicine* indicated that 7-keto DHEA was safe for human consumption in doses of 200 mg per day for up to four weeks. The safety of internal use beyond four weeks is not known.[105]

Osteoporosis

Osteoporosis—which means "porous bones"—is a progressive loss of bone mass that leads to decreased bone density. Expecting to instantly reverse everything that has been happening in your body may be unrealistic. Remember, it has taken years and probably decades for your bones to degenerate. However, you can restore your bones with wonderful supplements that provide the nutrients you need to battle and win over osteoporosis.

Eating correctly and taking supplements is a long-term process. Be persistent—not impatient. Don't get discouraged if you feel that you are not moving along quickly enough. Start your journey toward feeling better by taking these significant supplements.

A good multivitamin

The foundation of a good supplement program always starts with a comprehensive multivitamin. Adequate doses of many of the nutrients I am about to discuss are found in a good multivitamin.

Calcium

This supplement's effectiveness can be reduced by whole grains containing phytic acid, which may reduce the absorption of calcium and other minerals. It is actually best to take calcium supplements after meals because hydrochloric acid in the stomach is increased with food and helps calcium absorption.

The first part of the small intestines, called the duodenum, is the main place where it is absorbed. Don't take all of your calcium at one time since your body can absorb only about 500 mg of calcium at one time.

This rate of calcium absorption can dip down as low as only 5 percent for calcium carbonate, if you are a postmenopausal woman who is lacking hydrochloric acid. You could actually be taking in 1,500 mg of calcium carbonate a day and only absorbing 75 mg, which is only 5 percent. You can see by the loss of calcium daily through non-absorption that taking 1,500 mg can still result in significant bone loss.

In addition, I do not recommend some sources of calcium. These include oyster shell since it may contain significant amounts of lead. Dolomite also may contain relatively high amounts of lead. So, be careful when buying calcium.

A chelated form of calcium, which is bound to an amino acid such as calcium citrate, calcium aspartate, or calcium fumarate, is more easily absorbed.

Calcium hydroxyapatite, a form of calcium that is derived from bone, is absorbed fairly well. Because it comes from bone meal, it contains all the different minerals in their natural state. However, be careful not to purchase just any brand, for some also can contain lead. Even though the daily value of calcium is 1,200 mg a day for women over fifty, I now recommend that women take in only 200–250 mg of chelated calcium or calcium hydroxyapatite three times a day. Remember not to take too much calcium. A recent study showed that calcium supplementation may increase the risk of heart attack.[106] Taking vitamin K_2 100 mcg a day with calcium has been shown to keep calcium in the bones rather than the arteries.[107]

Calcium absorption is dependent upon vitamin D as well as bile, bile salts, and dietary fat. Patients with a low amount of stomach acid (a fairly common occurrence in postmenopausal women) need to take a well-absorbed calcium, such as chelated calcium, and not calcium carbonate. A chelated calcium does not need hydrochloric acid to be absorbed. I recommend a supplement that contains 200–250 mg of chelated calcium and about 100 mg of chelated magnesium, and take one with each meal, or three times per day. These can be found at most health food stores.

Vitamin D

This is a fat-soluble vitamin that is manufactured in our skin when it comes in contact with the sun's ultraviolet rays. Vitamin D is important for bone health. As I mentioned earlier, since it is difficult to get vitamin D from foods and most Americans are not exposed to adequate sunlight, I recommend vitamin D supplements. I typically recommend 2,000 IU per day for most patients, but I may increase the dose to 5,000–10,000 IU per day for a few months until the vitamin D level reaches the optimal range, which is 50–80 ng/ml.

Even though cod liver oil is high in vitamin D, it also contains significant amounts of vitamin A. Studies have shown that high doses of vitamin A may increase your risk of a fracture. For example, some studies have shown that increased intake of vitamin A (retinol form) can increase your risk of a fracture by 40 percent.[108] For this reason, I do not recommend cod liver oil to patients with osteoporosis or osteopenia.

Strict vegetarians who do not eat any meat, eggs, or milk products and who do not get adequate sun exposure should take a supplement with at least 1,000–2,000 IU or higher daily, depending on their vitamin D_3 blood test.

Magnesium

This mineral helps increase the absorption of calcium in your diet, and it also helps your bones retain or hold on to the calcium. Without adequate amounts of magnesium, you are more prone to losing bone more rapidly.

The standard American diet provides inadequate amounts of magnesium. Caffeine, sugar, alcohol, and soft drinks cause magnesium to be depleted.

Magnesium is found naturally in dark green vegetables, nuts, seeds, and legumes, as well as whole grains such as whole wheat. Chlorophyll is the green pigment in plants, and the central atom of the chlorophyll is magnesium. Therefore, high-chlorophyll products are excellent sources of magnesium.

Because it can be hard to get enough magnesium from your diet, I recommend supplementing a balanced diet with a good comprehensive multivitamin, which will contain approximately 400 mg of magnesium. If you take calcium supplements, keep in mind that most calcium supplements do not contain magnesium, and calcium should be balanced with magnesium in approximately a two-to-one ratio.[109] In other words, if you consume 600 mg of calcium a day, you should take approximately 300 mg of magnesium a day.

An acidic environment in the stomach is required for magnesium to be adequately absorbed. Eating a diet high in fats, proteins, or phosphorus also may hinder magnesium absorption. Similar to calcium, only about 40 percent of the magnesium that we consume is absorbed.[110] Chelated magnesium is the most absorbable form of magnesium, such as magnesium malate, magnesium asparate, or magnesium citrate. Magnesium salt, such as magnesium oxide and magnesium carbonate, is not nearly as easily absorbed as chelated varieties.

Other important nutrients

There are many nutrients that are very important for bone health and for reversing osteoporosis. In addition to calcium, magnesium, and vitamin D_3, which I have just discussed, vitamin K_2, boron, vitamin B_6, vitamin B_{12}, folic acid, zinc, copper, vitamin C, potassium, phosphorus, manganese, silica, silicon, and strontium are important. Fortunately most of these nutrients can be obtained in a good comprehensive multivitamin. Here is some additional information about some of these nutrients and their effect on bone health.

Vitamin K_2

It is interesting to note that as we age, our bones lose calcium and become brittle, but our arteries typically become calcified. However, vitamin K_2 is able to regulate calcium metabolism by keeping calcium in the bones and out of our arteries. Vitamin K is found in two different forms in nature: vitamin K_1, which is found in green leafy vegetables and is important in blood clotting, and the lesser-known vitamin K_2, which is found in egg yolks, organ meats, and dairy. Most physicians discourage patients from eating organ meats and eggs since they are both high in cholesterol, and as a result most Americans do not consume enough vitamin K_2.

However, in certain areas of Japan, a staple dish of fermented soybeans called "natto" is commonly eaten a few times a week and is very rich in vitamin K_2. The Japanese people who consume this dish typically have much higher blood levels of vitamin K_2 and significantly fewer occurrences of osteoporosis and bone fractures.[111] Vitamin K_2 is frequently prescribed for osteoporosis in Japan.[112]

Vitamin K_2 helps increase the building of bones and decrease bone loss. If you take Coumadin, use of vitamin K_2 should be discussed with your doctor. For treating osteoporosis, I typically recommend at least 100 mcg per day, and sometimes I may recommend 1,000 mcg or more per day.

The B-vitamin family

A good comprehensive multivitamin will contain B vitamins, folic acid, vitamin B_6, and vitamin B_{12} in doses that lower levels of the toxic amino acid homocysteine. High levels of the toxic amino acid homocysteine are associated with fractures in patients with osteoporosis. It is very important to have your homocysteine level checked and to lower it to a level less than 10 micromoles per liter.

I recommend approximately 800 mcg per day of folic acid, approximately 100–500 mcg per day of vitamin B_{12}, and approximately 10–20 mg per day of B_6 if one has elevated homocysteine levels.

Be sure to have your physician check your homocysteine level a few months after starting your multivitamin, and if it is still elevated a few months later, then I recommend adding 1,000 mg of trimethylglycine (also known as TMG) once or twice a day and 1–5 mg of methyltetrahydrofolate (MTHF) a day, which is the active form of folic acid.

Many doctors do not check homocysteine levels when diagnosing or treating osteoporosis, so be sure to ask your doctor about this very important lab test.

Boron

Boron is a mineral that is needed in trace amounts for healthy bones and is also necessary for the metabolism of calcium, phosphorus, and magnesium. A good comprehensive multivitamin will contain adequate amounts of boron, which is 2–3 mg a day.

Boron also helps maximize the activity of estrogen and vitamin D in bone. Boron is involved in an enzyme reaction in the kidneys, where vitamin D is converted to its most powerful bone-building form. Boron is also needed for the conversion of estrogen to its most powerful bone-building form, which is 17 beta-estradiol. Good food sources of boron are leafy green vegetables, legumes, nuts, apples, and pears.[113]

Strontium

Most people think of strontium as the toxic strontium 90, a toxic radioactive component of nuclear fallout and associated with increased risk of cancer. However, stable strontium is nonradioactive, nontoxic, and a trace mineral. It is also one of the most effective supplements found for the treatment of osteoporosis. Taking stable strontium can gradually eliminate radioactive strontium from the body. Strontium, found in seawater, is one of the most abundant trace minerals on earth. Strontium also has been used safely for more than one hundred years.[114]

One study involved 1,649 postmenopausal women with osteoporosis who received for three years either 680 mg of strontium a day or a placebo. The main bone mineral density of the lumbar spine increased in the strontium group by an average of 14.4 percent after three years. Strontium, when compared with the placebo, decreased the incidence of vertebral fractures by 49 percent after one year and by 41 percent after three years.[115]

Taking doses of strontium up to 1.7 g a day is a safe and effective way to treat osteoporosis. However, doses of 680 mg per day may be all that is needed to reverse osteoporosis. You also can boost your strontium intake by consuming spices, seafood, whole grains, root and leafy vegetables, and legumes.[116] Strontium needs to be taken on an empty stomach. I usually recommend strontium 680 mg one or two capsules a day on an empty stomach.

Silicon

Silicon is also important for bone strength. It is found in high amounts in wheat, oat, and rice bran. It also is found in alfalfa and in the herb horsetail. Dark green vegetables, avocados, onions, and strawberries also contain silicon. This substance helps restore and strengthen bones by strengthening the connective tissue collagen, which is at the matrix of the bone. I usually recommend silicon 30 mg once or twice a day.

Premenstrual Syndrome (PMS)

You may believe there aren't natural methods for relieving the symptoms of mood swings, PMS, depression, cramping, and monthly discomfort, but that isn't true. Vitamins and minerals are important for hormonal balance, and taking them will help restore your body back to this balance. But if you're like many of us, looking at health food and grocery store shelves lined with bottles of vitamins and other supplements can leave you feeling a little mystified. Here is some practical and easy information about some of these powerful natural substances that can have you feeling better in no time.

Supplements for mood swings and PMS

Consider taking these supplements.

A comprehensive multivitamin/multimineral

Improve your PMS and premenopause symptoms with zinc and a comprehensive multivitamin including vitamin B_6, all the other B-complex vitamins, and 400 mg per day of magnesium. These nutrients help balance the hormones in the body. Take a good comprehensive multivitamin one to two times a day.

Bioidentical progesterone cream

Bioidentical progesterone cream can help balance your hormones and reduce PMS symptoms. It also helps reduce the pain of tender, swollen breasts. Progesterone helps calm the mind and relieve mood swings and irritability.

In addition, most premenopausal women are very often estrogen dominant. Those high estrogen levels can cause you to crave carbohydrates and sugars and make you gain weight. You can sometimes balance the estrogen levels by supplementing with natural progesterone cream. Use 3 percent progesterone cream. Apply one to two pumps once or twice a day, especially from days twelve through twenty-six in the menstrual cycle. Day one is the first day of the menstrual period. For tender, swollen breasts, rub the cream directly on breasts.

Flaxseed

Take 2–3 tablespoons of flaxseed one to three times a day. Flaxseed contain fatty acids, which have been shown to help control side effects of PMS.[117]

Vitamin E

Vitamin E can help reduce breast tenderness. If this is an ongoing severe problem, you also may need to have your dosage of birth control medication decreased or eliminated. Take 400–800 IU daily to help decrease breast tenderness. Purchase natural vitamin E, which contains all eight forms of vitamin E.

Chasteberry

For irregular periods, the herb chasteberry, which is also called vitex, can usually help. This herb actually helps stimulate the hypothalamus to increase the luteinizing hormone (LH). This, in turn, may help stimulate the production of progesterone. Take 200–225 mg of a standardized extract of vitex a day, or drink chasteberry tea.

Gamma-linolenic acid (GLA)

GLA is found in evening primrose oil, borage oil, and black currant oil. GLA may be helpful in controlling cyclic breast tenderness. The body also needs adequate amounts of B_6, magnesium, and zinc in order to make enough of its own GLA, whish is usually found in a comprehensive multivitamin.

The usual dose of GLA is 200–400 mg a day. Or you may take

approximately 4 g of evening primrose oil a day or about 2 g of borage oil a day. Be patient, however, for it may take a few months to notice the benefits of this.

Dong quai

This is commonly recommended for menstrual cramps, PMS, and hot flashes. It may be taken in capsules, tablets, tinctures, or teas. A common dose is 3 g a day. It is found in most health food stores.

Black cohosh

Black cohosh has been used for over forty years. It helps decrease many of the symptoms of perimenopause and menopause, including hot flashes, depression, and insomnia. Though traditionally taken for menopause or perimenopause, this supplement also may be helpful for PMS symptoms. The black cohosh product called Remifemin is a German product and is of very high quality. Take one tablet twice a day.

Help for excessive bleeding

If your PMS is accompanied by heavy bleeding, get a pelvic ultrasound to rule out uterine fibroids. These are commonly associated with heavy bleeding. To help control heavy bleeding, you usually will need a stronger natural progesterone cream, such as 6 or 10 percent.

- Use 60–100 mg of progesterone cream twice a day on days twelve through twenty-six to better control heavy bleeding.
- Take two to three tablespoons of ground flaxseed two to three times a day in a smoothie or in water.
- Taking 500–1,000 mg of vitamin C with bioflavonoids three times a day may help decrease blood loss from heavy menstruation.
- If heavy bleeding continues, have a complete blood count taken together with a serum iron and ferritin level blood test to see if you need an iron supplement. You may need to supplement with iron to prevent or to treat iron-deficiency anemia and follow up with your physician.

Loss of sex drive

Estrogen dominance not only will cause you to gain weight, but it will often cause a loss of sex drive. As excess estrogen may suppress sex drive, the hormones progesterone and testosterone usually will increase it. That's why I often place PMS sufferers who are experiencing a loss of sex drive on both bioidentical progesterone cream and bioidentical testosterone cream. This usually will help balance your estrogen and dramatically improve your sex drive. I use a very small dose of testosterone cream and monitor testosterone levels to avoid side effects.

Stress-busting solutions

Stress usually plays a major role in the symptoms of PMS and premenopause. Many, if not most, of the symptoms of premenopause are related to stressed adrenal glands. Many women's lives are so busy with their work, home, children, husband, church, and social activities that they end up having too little time left to take care of themselves.

If this sounds like you, your busy, stressed-out lifestyle can cause your body's levels of epinephrine and cortisol to become elevated. Higher levels of cortisol will actually lead to decreased levels of progesterone. Elevated cortisol levels can result in weight gain, memory loss, blood sugar changes, insomnia, irritability, and depression. Eventually your adrenal glands can get so worn out that you may develop chronic fatigue, low blood pressure, allergies, low metabolic rate with cold hands and cold feet, depression, irregular periods, and recurring infections. Remember that no supplement is as important as adequate sleep, rest, and relaxation. Refer to the section on adrenal fatigue for supplements.

Dehydroepiandrosterone (DHEA) and pregnenolone

I normally place women on either DHEA, 10–25 mg once or twice a day, or pregnenolone, 30 mg a day. Pregnenolone is the raw material for making progesterone.

If you are pregnant, or plan on becoming pregnant, stop *all* supplements and consult your physician.

Prostate Disorders

If you are battling prostate disease, you are in a war with a dangerous enemy. Though you are not at war against flesh and blood warriors, your foe is as insidious and destructive as any armed enemy in combat. Your diet is important to control prostate disorder. Read my book *Let Food Be Your Medicine*, and follow the dietary suggestions for preventing cancer. Supplements are important as well.

Supplements can arm your body with what it needs for a frontal attack against the source of prostate cancer and benign prostatic hypertrophy (BPH). Taking the right supplements can help you reduce dramatically your risk of developing prostate disease. Additionally, supplements have the ability to assist your body's battle in reversing prostate disease even after it is diagnosed.

Antioxidants

Target cancer-causing free radicals in your body with antioxidants. Antioxidants are powerfully effective in preventing prostate cancer and keeping it from becoming active and spreading when it resides in a dormant state.

In a Finnish study called the Alpha-Tocopherol, Beta-Carotene Cancer Prevention (ATBC) trial, men taking the antioxidant vitamin E experienced a 40 percent decreased death rate from prostate cancer when compared with those who didn't take antioxidants. In addition to that, the men also had a 30 percent decreased risk of being diagnosed with prostate cancer. Here's a list of some powerful antioxidants and other supplements you should take every day.

Comprehensive vitamin E

Vitamin E is fat soluble, which means it is particularly effective in reaching fatty tissues, such as those found in the prostate. Take at least 400–800 IU per day, and check the label to be sure it contains all eight forms of vitamin E and especially gamma toctorienol and gamma tocopherols. A study found that gamma tocotrienol was effective in targeting prostate cancer stem cells.

Selenium

This power-packed antioxidant is vital for your cancer-busting arsenal. It has been shown that men who have the lowest levels of selenium in their bloodstream were also 50 percent more likely to develop prostate cancer, whereas those with the highest levels were 50 percent less likely to develop prostate cancer.

Selenium and a comprehensive vitamin E complement each other amazingly well. Together they form a powerful shield of antioxidant protection against prostate cancer. Take at least 100–200 mcg of selenium daily.

Vitamin D

Vitamin D has long been seen as a natural cancer protector. A few years ago, scientists discovered that American men who lived in the northern states experienced higher mortality rates from prostate cancer than those from the South. These scientists surmised that the leading factor for this difference was vitamin D because sunlight exposure increases the production of vitamin D in the body. Those men living in the southern states would potentially have greater exposure to sunlight than those living farther north.

In addition, a lack of vitamin D is considered a major reason for the increased rates of prostate cancer among African American men because their darker skin absorbs less sunlight, resulting in lower levels of vitamin D.

The best way to increase your vitamin D is to spend more time out of doors in the sunlight; fifteen to twenty minutes daily at noontime is best. If you're trapped in an office all day, try eating your lunch at a picnic table outdoors. I put most of my patients on 2,000 IU of vitamin D a day, but some patients require 5,000 IU or more a day in order to get their vitamin D levels in the optimal range, which is 50–80 ng/ml.

Curcumin

Curcumin, the valuable compound found in the spice turmeric, may help prevent or fight prostate cancer. It probably does this because curcumin inhibits the cyclooxygenase-2 (COX-2) enzyme that promotes inflammation. Research has shown that curcumin can remove ten different cancer-causing factors. It:

- Blocks nuclear factor-kappaB, a molecule causing inflammation
- Disrupts the body's production of advanced glycation end products, which cause inflammation
- Enhances the control of replication of cells
- Encourages cell death in cancer cells that are quickly reproducing
- Increases the vulnerability of tumors
- Increases the death of cancer cells by regulating pathways of tumor suppressors
- Limits the invasiveness of tumors
- Blocks "pathways to penetration of tissue"
- Reduces blood supply of tumors
- Limits the ability of cancer to spread[118]

Curcumin also can be taken in supplement form. It is an antioxidant several times more powerful than vitamin E. Piperine, a compound found in pepper, increases its absorption. Because of this and the incredible health benefits of curcumin for multiple diseases, I suggest you have 500–1,000 mg of turmeric once or twice a day in a supplement that also includes piperine to increase its effectiveness.

Supplement strategies for benign prostatic hypertrophy (BPH)

In addition to preventing and treating cancer, supplements are a powerful part of your health strategy for BPH, an enlarged prostate gland.

Saw palmetto

This powerful prostate-healing herb is made from the berries of the saw palmetto plant, which is found in my home state of Florida. Saw palmetto has been recognized as an effective treatment for BPH in many European countries.

Symptoms of BPH usually improve in about four to six weeks in two-thirds of men who take saw palmetto. Some studies have shown that saw palmetto is as effective as the medication Proscar, and with far fewer side effects.

The standard dose of saw palmetto is 160 mg twice a day. However, you may increase this to 320 mg twice a day after six weeks if your symptoms have not improved.

Before you begin taking saw palmetto, it's important to have your doctor give you a digital rectal exam and a prostate-specific antigen (PSA) test to rule out prostate cancer. In addition, be sure to inform your doctor in future visits that you are taking saw palmetto before having a PSA screening since it may lower your PSA level.

Beta-sitosterol

This is probably the most important supplement you can take for BPH. Beta-sitosterol is a powerful plant nutrient used in Germany for more than twenty years for treating benign prostatic hypertrophy. Some plants, such as rice bran, soybeans, and wheat germ, contain particularly high levels of beta-sitosterol. I recommend 400–800 mg of beta-sitosterol two times a day.

Sitosterol inhibits the production of inflammatory prostaglandins, which, in turn, lowers prostate congestion. Studies have shown that beta-sitosterol can improve urinary symptoms related to prostate disorders. Common in Europe, this supplement is said to help the prostate by reducing swelling.[119]

Pygeum africanum

Another powerful herb that improves the symptoms of BPH is *pygeum africanum*, made from an evergreen tree that is native to Africa. The bark contains active sterols and fatty acids, and *pygeum africanum* also actually contains beta-sitosterol. However, studies indicate that saw palmetto is more effective. The standard dosage of *pygeum africanum* is 100 mg of the standardized extract twice a day.

Nettle root

Another herb effective in the treatment of BPH is nettle root. This herb often is combined with saw palmetto and *pygeum africanum* to treat BPH. Take 120 mg twice a day.

Zinc

Getting enough zinc is vital for prostate health, especially if you have BPH. Prostate secretions contain high concentrations of zinc. Therefore, zinc plays an important role in healthy prostate functioning.

Take 50–75 mg of chelated zinc such as zinc citrate in divided doses. Repeat the zinc tally test after a month of taking supplements. Place a teaspoon of zinc sulfate on your tongue, and hold it in your mouth for five seconds. If you still cannot taste the zinc, which has a bitter flavor, then you are probably not absorbing enough of it into your system. You may need to try a liquid form of this supplement.

Crila

Crila is from a rare herb that is said to have been used for royalty in Vietnam for centuries to treat symptoms of prostate disorders. Now it is used as a new supplement for BPH. It is from an herb grown in Vietnam that contains crinum latifolium. Studies have shown that this supplement has incredible results in treating those with prostate disorders. One hundred fifty-seven men took Crila for prostate health; 140 of them had noticeable improvements in only two weeks. For best results, it needs to be taken for eight weeks.[120] One should do a loading phase for two months of four to six capsules containing 3 g of Crila twice a day and then just two capsules a day thereafter.

SKIN DISORDERS

Supplements are a powerful way to be sure that your body's largest organ, your skin, is getting all that it needs to battle skin disorders. In addition, supplement power can help support healing and restore the beauty of normal skin function. The skin is usually a reflection of the gastrointestinal (GI) tract, and most patients with psoriasis have inflammation in their GI tract. The inflammation may be due to food sensitivities, food allergies, yeast overgrowth, dysbiosis, parasites, etc. I always perform an antigen leukocyte cellular antibody test (ALCAT) to identify food sensitivities as well as GI tests to identify pathogens and then treat them accordingly.

Supplements for psoriasis and eczema

As you begin your supplement program, it will be very helpful to test for polyamines, those toxic compounds formed in the GI tract as a result of incomplete digestion of protein. You can be tested for polyamines through a simple urine test, the indican test. It will confirm the need to lower your level of polyamines, which you can do through diet and taking proper supplements.

Fish oil (omega-3 fatty acids)

Fish oil prevents the production of arachidonic acid, a major culprit in psoriasis and eczema. Supplementing omega-3 fatty acids may be one of the most important things you can do for healing your skin. Also, make sure the fish oil is not rancid, as many that are in health food stores can be. I usually start patients on one EPA/DHA supplement that contains 1,000 mg of EPA/DHA. I usually recommend 1,000–2,000 mg twice a day.

Krill with astaxanthin

Krill is a fatty acid that contains astaxanthin naturally. Astaxanthin is an antioxidant found in algae. It protects cells in the body from free radicals, including cells in the brain, heart, kidneys, and more. Astaxanthin actually increases the effectiveness of fatty acids. This is a powerful supplement for reducing inflammation.[121]

A comprehensive multivitamin

The rapid cell division in skin disorders can create nutritional deficiencies. In addition, patients with skin disorders usually have low levels of zinc and vitamin A, as well as deficiencies of B vitamins, selenium, chromium, vitamin E, and other antioxidants. A comprehensive multivitamin will help correct any vitamin and mineral deficiencies. See appendix A.

L-glutamine

Most of the patients that I see with psoriasis have impaired intestinal permeability. L-glutamine is an amino acid that improves intestinal permeability. It also feeds the cells of the small intestines. I recommend taking 500–1,000 mg of L-glutamine thirty minutes before eating your meals.

Fiber

Another very important supplement for helping psoriasis is fiber, which helps bind the toxins *and* excrete them in the feces, thus reducing the body's overall toxic burden. The two main types of fiber are soluble and insoluble. Excessive amounts of soluble fiber, such as beans, psyllium seeds, and peas and legumes can actually lead to an overgrowth of intestinal bacteria, and thus may actually worsen psoriasis.

Insoluble fiber, on the other hand, helps inactivate many of the intestinal toxins. It also helps prevent harmful bacteria and parasites from attaching themselves to the wall of your intestines by acting like a sweeping broom. An excellent insoluble fiber found in health food stores, microcrystalline cellulose, does not contain any wheat products and tends to be tolerated by those with sensitive GI tracts.

I usually recommend starting with one teaspoon of fiber twice a day, usually mixed with water or a protein drink, and then gradually increasing up to one tablespoon twice a day.

Glutathione-boosting supplement

As has previously been stated, glutathione is the most important antioxidant in the body. It serves as a detoxifier of the body, neutralizing toxins and heavy metals as well as quenching free radicals. All of this has been shown to prevent damage to our skin and help heal our GI tract. RiboCeine is the best way to boost the glutathione in your body. I recommend RiboCeine

(MaxOne) one to two capsules twice a day or N-acetyl cysteine 500 mg one to two capsules twice a day.

Probiotics

Studies still need to be done, but early research shows that probiotics, or good bacteria, may help lessen the severity of skin disorders such as eczema. There are two primary types of probiotics: lactobacillus and bifidobacterium. I would recommend 50–200 billion colony-forming units of a diversity of multiple strains of different probiotics in the morning upon awakening.

Herbal teas

Certain herbal teas, such as slippery elm bark tea and saffron tea, are highly recommended for treating psoriasis. Dr. John O. A. Pagano, who has successfully treated many patients with severe cases of psoriasis, recommends drinking saffron tea before bedtime.[122] Place a quarter of a teaspoon of saffron tea in a cup, and then pour boiling water over it. After letting it stand for fifteen to thirty minutes, strain it and drink it. I recommend adding a small amount of liquid stevia to taste.

Dr. Pagano also recommends a cup of slippery elm bark tea in the early morning, approximately thirty minutes prior to breakfast. Make it fresh each time. He recommends placing a quarter of a teaspoon of slippery elm bark powder in a cup of warm water and letting it stand for about fifteen minutes prior to drinking it. Do not strain the slippery elm tea; it is a mucilage, which soothes inflamed mucous membranes of the bowels and is beneficial for most inflammatory conditions of the GI tract. Slippery elm tea can be taken two to three times a day.

Healing supplements for acne

I recommend that my patients with acne stop all gluten and follow my anti-inflammatory diet in my book *Let Food Be Your Medicine*.

Benzoyl peroxide

A very inexpensive and effective treatment for acne is benzoyl peroxide, which can be purchased over the counter at your pharmacy. Benzoyl peroxide is an oxidizing agent that dries and peels the skin; it also helps loosen impactions.

For any acne treatment to be successful, the skin must become dry and peel. Expect it to become irritated. This means the medicine or treatment is penetrating into the pores and helping to break up and remove the impactions, releasing oxygen that kills the bacteria. Benzoyl peroxide comes in three different strengths: 2.5 percent, 5 percent, and 10 percent.

For sensitive skin, start with the 2.5 percent strength once or twice a day. After a few weeks, you can increase the strength to the 5 percent. For normal skin, start with the 5 percent strength twice a day, and after a few weeks, gradually increase it to 10 percent. Do not purchase benzoyl peroxide products that contain oil since they are less effective.

Rub benzoyl peroxide everywhere acne occurs, such as the nose, cheeks, chin, forehead, and possibly the jaw line, as well as the back and chest. Avoid the area around the eyes, and also avoid the corner of the mouth and the area under the nostrils.

If your skin becomes too irritated, red, and inflamed, simply lay off the benzoyl peroxide for a few days and give your skin a break. Don't start using moisturizers. Expect mild, but not severe, irritation.

I advise my patients to avoid oral antibiotics, which can cause candida overgrowth. Topically applied antibiotic lotions may be effective in some individuals, however.

Vitamin A

Vitamin A is a very healing supplement for acne, as it normalizes the growth of skin cells and helps remove impactions and prevent new ones from developing. However, vitamin A is potentially toxic at high doses, with serious side effects. Therefore, I do not recommend taking more than 10,000 IU per day or 5,000 IU daily for pregnant women.

I recommend a topical vitamin A prescription known as Retin-A (tretinoin). Besides providing the healing properties of vitamin A, the topical application will ensure that you avoid negative side effects caused by high doses of oral vitamin A. Use Retin-A only once a day, in the evening, after washing your face. Overuse can be very irritating to your skin. If your skin gets red and irritated, stop the Retin-A for a few days and try using it every other day. An excellent medication for acne is Epiduo, which combines benzoyl peroxide with tretinoin and is prescribed by a medical doctor.

Also, while using this product, avoid or dramatically limit sun exposure since Retin-A makes the skin more prone to sunburn. You can ask your family doctor or dermatologist to prescribe Retin-A gel or Epiduo.

Zinc

A very important nutrient for treatment of acne is zinc. A zinc supplement may help decrease the inflammation in those with severe acne. I recommend zinc picolinate or zinc citrate approximately 50 mg a day.

Probiotics

Many patients with acne have been over-prescribed oral antibiotics, which kill the friendly bacteria in the intestinal tract. Probiotics, or beneficial bacteria, must be replaced for a few months. I recommend probiotics that have multiple strains and have 50–200 billion colony-forming units.

Fiber

Taking a fiber supplement in the form of ground flaxseed, chia seeds, psyllium, or any other type of soluble fiber every day will be helpful, binding testosterone as well as other hormones in the GI tract and eliminating them from the body. That's important for acne because too much testosterone in the body, as is the case of many teens, triggers acne. If you are a female with severe acne, ask your doctor to check your androgenic hormones, including testosterone, total and free. If testosterone levels are high, you may need the medication Aldactone, which is a diuretic that lowers testosterone levels. Many times one tablespoon of chia seeds taken twice a day will lower testosterone levels and improve acne.

It's also important to take a fiber supplement daily to assure regular bowel movements. Many individuals with acne are constipated. Drinking two quarts of filtered water a day and taking a fiber supplement may dramatically improve acne conditions.

Azelaic acid

Azelaic acid is a natural product that is very effective for all forms of acne. It removes the impaction caused by the dead cells within the pore, and it has an antibacterial effect. Creams containing 20 percent azelaic acid have been shown to produce results equal to those of benzoyl peroxide, Retin-A, and oral tetracycline.[123]

Azelaic acid should be applied to all acne-prone areas twice a day. I recommend choosing to use either benzoyl peroxide or azelaic acid, but not both. Expect to see results after using it for one month. You can ask your doctor to prescribe azelaic acid, or you may find it in some health food stores.

Alpha hydroxy acids (AHA)

Alpha hydroxy acids, such as glycolic acid, are fruit acids that can remove dead skin cells and stimulate the cells in the epidermis to produce new cells, which, interestingly, do not usually cause the impactions that lead to acne. Once the dead skin cells are removed with this product, the benzoyl peroxide, Retin-A, or azelaic acid will actually work better.

A dermatologist or esthetician can administer a chemical peel containing these acids, or you can purchase alpha hydroxy acids or glycolic acid at most cosmetic counters. Just make sure that those cosmetic preparations do not contain any oils or other ingredients that can produce a breakout.

SLEEP DISORDERS

The benefits to your body and mind of plenty of restful sleep cannot be measured. Sleep is vital to your health and well-being, allowing you to recharge your mind and body, and allowing your body to recuperate and restore itself from exhaustion.

One way to walk in wisdom is to understand good stewardship of your own health by providing your body with all it needs for proper sleep. In addition, learn what nutrients, herbs, and other supplements can help.

Supplementing your diet with vitamins, minerals, herbs, amino acids, and other supplements can dramatically impact many sleep disorders. So let's take a look at a program of supplementation that will make you wiser about helping your body to sleep.

To begin a supplementation program, be sure that your body has all the vitamins and minerals it needs to function at optimal levels. Start with a good comprehensive multivitamin/multimineral supplement. I strongly recommend one that contains adequate levels of B vitamins, magnesium, and trace minerals. This will provide optimal nutritional supplementation for a good night's sleep.

Insomnia

Several special herbs and other supplements are especially effective in helping you sleep. However, you will find that supplementing with magnesium, melatonin, certain amino acids, herbs, or hormones at bedtime, or drinking teas, is very effective; also, these teas and supplements are nonaddictive, unlike most medications for sleep. Herbs and supplements for sleep are usually used on a short-term basis unless you have anxiety, depression, or a deficiency in melatonin or certain calming neurotransmitters.

Let's look at some of these helpful supplements.

Melatonin

Melatonin is a hormone produced by a small gland called the pineal gland, in the brain. Melatonin helps regulate sleep and wake cycles, or circadian rhythms. Usually melatonin begins to rise in the evening and remains high for most of the night and then decreases in the early morning. Melatonin production is affected by light. As a person ages, melatonin levels decline.

Older adults typically produce very small amounts of melatonin or none at all. Studies suggest that melatonin induces sleep without suppressing rapid eye movement (REM) or dream sleep, whereas most sleep meds suppress REM sleep.[124]

Melatonin works best if the patient's melatonin levels are low. Children generally have normal levels of melatonin; therefore, supplementation with melatonin in children usually is ineffective. However, in adults, especially the elderly, it may be very effective in treating insomnia and is excellent in treating jet lag. It is also usually very effective for those who work the night shift.

The main side effect of melatonin is sleepiness, which is good; however, other potential side effects include vivid dreams, morning grogginess, and headaches. The recommended dose of melatonin is typically 1–6 mg at bedtime. However, some patients may need up to 20 mg at nighttime. I recommend a melatonin lozenge since it dissolves in the mouth and seems to work better for most patients. I start my patients on a low dose and gradually increase the dose until the patient is sleeping well.

I also commonly continue melatonin with other natural sleep aids that you will be learning about soon. Remember, melatonin as well as other sleep aids work best when your life is conducive to sleeping well.

L-tryptophan and 5-hydroxytryptophan (5-HTP)

I commonly place patients with insomnia on melatonin and the amino acid L-tryptophan or 5-HTP. L-tryptophan improves sleep normalcy and increases stage four sleep (the most restorative stage of sleep). It also has been shown to improve obstructive sleep apnea in many patients, and it does not decrease cognitive performance.

Both L-tryptophan and its metabolite 5-HTP are used to increase serotonin levels in the brain. Serotonin is a neurotransmitter in the brain that promotes restful sleep and well-being as well as satiety.

However, when serotonin levels are low in the brain, you are more prone to experience insomnia. Serotonin levels also are increased by ingesting carbohydrates. When carbohydrates such as pasta are ingested with L-tryptophan or 5-HTP, the elevated insulin level increases the removal of other amino acids that compete with tryptophan and 5-HTP for transport into the brain. Carbohydrates also tend to increase the sedative effects of 5-HTP and tryptophan.

I recommend vitamin B_6, niacin, and magnesium, which serve as cofactors in the conversion of L-tryptophan and 5-HTP to serotonin. I usually recommend simply taking either 1,000–2,000 mg of L-tryptophan or 100–300 mg of 5-HTP at bedtime. In addition, I recommend a comprehensive multivitamin that contains adequate amounts of vitamin B_6, niacin, and magnesium, which helps convert L-tryptophan and 5-HTP to serotonin. Also, I usually have the patients take their L-tryptophan or 5-HTP with a food that is high in carbohydrates and low in protein, such as a Fiber One bar or, if not overweight, a serving of brown rice pasta.

L-theanine and gamma-aminobutyric acid (GABA)

I have found that most patients with insomnia are under excessive stress and may be suffering from anxiety and depression. Excessive stress, anxiety, and depression are usually associated with elevated cortisol levels, especially at night. Elevated stress hormones, especially cortisol, eventually disrupt brain chemistry, causing imbalances in neurotransmitters, including serotonin, dopamine, norepinephrine, and GABA, as well as other brain chemicals.

However, the amino acid L-theanine crosses the blood-brain barrier and is able to suppress stress hormones, including cortisol. L-theanine is one of the natural chemicals found in green tea and helps decrease stress and anxiety. It also helps the body produce other calming neurotransmitters, including GABA, serotonin, and dopamine. In Japan, L-theanine is usually added to sodas and chewing gum to provide a relaxing and soothing effect.[125]

I find that L-theanine typically works better with the amino acid GABA. GABA is also a calming neurotransmitter in the brain that has a soothing effect on the nervous system. L-theanine and GABA supplements taken with vitamin B_6 usually help calm the mind as well as lower the stress hormones and help you fall asleep. I usually recommend 200–400 mg of L-theanine with 500–1,000 mg of GABA at bedtime taken with a comprehensive multivitamin containing vitamin B_6. This combination also may be taken with melatonin and 5-HTP or L-tryptophan. For more information on GABA, please see *The New Bible Cure for Depression and Anxiety*.

Magnesium

We already know that adequate amounts of magnesium are needed to help convert L-tryptophan and 5-HTP to serotonin. There is also a close association between normal sleep architecture and magnesium. The excitatory neurotransmitter glutamate disrupts normal sleep architecture, causing insomnia, whereas the inhibitory neurotransmitter GABA usually improves sleep architecture. Magnesium is a mineral that helps decrease the glutamate activity in the brain while at the same time increasing the GABA activity in the brain. This usually helps improve sleep. Thus, magnesium is able to help many patients with insomnia issues.

I commonly recommend a magnesium powder, Neuro-Mag powder, to patients with insomnia. Simply taking one scoop of Neuro-Mag powder in four ounces of water or hot water as a tea at bedtime provides 144 mg of elemental magnesium, 500 mg of calcium lactate cluconate, and helps many of my patients fall asleep. Neuro-Mag contains magnesium threonate, which is a type of magnesium that readily crosses the blood-brain barrier, helping to induce sleep.

Sleep medications

I do not routinely recommend pharmaceutical medications for insomnia since they often have side effects. These include addiction or dependence upon the drug, rebound insomnia, and disrupting the normal architecture of sleep.

Rebound insomnia occurs when the insomnia becomes even worse after you go off the medication. Disrupting sleep architecture means that some sleep medications will make you fall asleep, but you will not spend adequate time in the deeper stages of sleep, such as stages three and four. Instead, most of your sleep time will be spent in the superficial stages, such as stages one and two.

Supplements for other sleep disorders

Since so many sleep disorders exist, let's look beyond insomnia to some supplements that help relieve the less-common sleep disorders.

Restless legs syndrome

If you are experiencing restless legs syndrome, get your doctor to test you to see if your body is low in iron. A test called a ferritin level blood test can measure the iron stores in your body.

If your ferritin level is low, supplementing with iron may relieve restless legs syndrome. Regular aerobic exercise, leg massages, and warm baths with Epsom salts, one to four cups in the bathwater, also can help relieve the symptoms of restless legs syndrome. Also, supplementation with magnesium at bedtime may help. I usually recommend the magnesium power Neuro-Mag, one scoop in four ounces of water at bedtime.

Periodic limb movement disorder

Periodic limb movement disorder is another movement disorder associated with insomnia. This involuntary disorder often causes repetitive, jerking twitches of the legs that last between one and three seconds. This twitching can wake up the sleeper or his or her spouse. Those with this disorder tend to feel quite drowsy throughout the day.

Here are some supplements that may help:

- 400 mg of magnesium in the form of magnesium citrate, magnesium aspartate, or magnesium glycinate, OR
- A scoop of NeuroMeg in four ounces of hot water at bedtime

In addition, taking a warm bath and adding one to four cups of Epsom salts to the bathwater may help.

STRESS

Chapter 4 talked about how stress depletes your body. People who are under excessive stress nearly always need to have an increase in the B vitamins (especially pantothenic acid, B_5), vitamin C, magnesium, zinc, copper, chromium, selenium, and vitamin E. One way to deal with the effects of stress is a sound supplement program including a comprehensive multivitamin.

The B Vitamins

The B vitamins (thiamine, riboflavin, niacin, pantothenic acid, folic acid, vitamin B_6, and vitamin B_{12}) are often called the "stress-relief vitamins." The

B-vitamin family provides the greatest benefit when supplemented together, such as a balanced B complex. Some B vitamins actually require other B vitamins for activation. The B vitamins are especially important for elderly individuals since they are not absorbed as well as a person ages. The B vitamins are associated primarily with brain and nervous system function.

Pantothenic acid (B_5)

Pantothenic acid is known as the "anti-stress" vitamin because it plays such a vital role in the production of adrenal hormones. A deficiency of pantothenic acid leads to a decreased resistance to stress.[126] Pantothenic acid provides critical support for the adrenal glands as it responds to stress, and adequate supplementation is very important for the health of adrenal glands in most people. I believe vitamin B_5 is the most important B vitamin for restoring and maintaining adrenal function. I typically place patients with adrenal fatigue on 500 mg two times a day.

Pantothenic acid can be found in salmon, yeast, vegetables, dairy, eggs, grains, and meat.

De-Stress Formula (DSF)

Stress and low adrenal function are often associated. Therefore, an adrenal glandular formula such as DSF or Drenamin can help stabilize the body's stress hormones. Take one to two tablets of DSF twice a day or two to three tablets of Drenamin in the morning and at lunch, to supply raw materials to help restore the adrenal function.

Dehydroepiandrosterone (DHEA)

DHEA is a hormone made naturally by your adrenal glands. When you are stressed and your adrenals are exhausted, often your supply of DHEA is low, which causes hormonal regulation in your entire body to suffer. You can replenish this vital hormone by taking it in supplement form. Take a small amount of DHEA. (Women usually need 10–25 mg a day; men, usually 25–50 mg a day.)

Adaptogens

An adaptogen is a substance that will help the body adapt to stress by balancing the adrenal gland's response to stress. The end result is that cortisol levels will be neither too high nor too low but will be balanced. One I recommend is *Rhodiola rosea,* an herb native to the mountainous regions of Asia, parts of Europe, and the Arctic. I recommend a product that uses a standardization of 2–3 percent rosavin, the active ingredient of *Rhodiola* used in clinical studies. The common dose is 200–600 mg three times a day. Others include ginseng, Korean ginseng, Siberian ginseng, ashwagandha, and magnolia bark. (See my book *Stress Less* for more information.)

THYROID DISORDERS

Feeling really tired lately? Perhaps you've gained weight or just can't seem to lose it no matter how hard you try. Are you cold all the time? Is your skin dryer than usual, or have you noticed that you seem extra thirsty or just achy? Maybe you've been kind of down, forgetful, constipated, or unusually irritable. If any of this sounds familiar, you may be a part of a hidden epidemic: hypothyroidism, or low-thyroid function. Most hyperthyroidism is due to autoimmune thyroiditis. I find that most of my patients with hypothyroidism are sensitive to gluten, and I take them off all gluten products. If caught early enough, some hypothyroid patients will not need thyroid medications. Please refer to my book *Let Food Be Your Medicine* for more information.

Hyperthyroid (Graves' disease) is so rare, I rarely treat patiens with this condition. That's why I'm not discussing it at length here. When I do have a patient with hyperthyroid, I prescribe Moducare and low-dose naltrexone.

Supplements for thyroid disorders

If you have a thyroid disorder, or a borderline thyroid disorder, supplements can help bring your body back into the right balance. Here are some supplements you may take.

A good multivitamin/multimineral. Your multivitamin should contain vitamin A, vitamin B_2, B_6, B_{12}, vitamin C, and zinc. Moderate amounts of these substances are essential for making thyroid hormone. Zinc is essential, but it also must be balanced with copper in a 10:1 ratio.

Selenium

Selenium, an important antioxidant, is one of the most important nutrients your body uses to convert thyroid hormone to meet your body's needs. Interestingly, Brazil nuts contain a whopping 840 mcg of selenium per ounce—twelve times as much as you need each day.

The daily value (DV) for selenium is 70 mcg, so check your label, as dosages can vary widely from brand to brand.

Dosage: take a multivitamin that contains at least 100 mcg of selenium, or take a selenium supplement. You may choose to simply eat a Brazil nut a day.

Low-dose naltrexone

Low-dose naltrexone is usually very beneficial for patients with autoimmune disorders. It has been used in higher doses (50 mg) for decades to treat patients addicted to heroin, other opiates, and alcohol. When one takes low-dose naltrexone at bedtime, it helps prevent overactivity of the immune system, which is the root cause of autoimmune disease. The usual dose is 1.5–4.5 mg at bedtime. This is prescribed by a medical doctor.

Moducare

Moducare is a blend of plant sterols and sterolins that work to restore, strengthen, and balance your body's immune system. Because they help balance the immune system, Moducare may prove effective in helping treat both Hashimoto's thyroiditis, the leading cause of hypothyroidism, and Graves' disease, the leading cause of hyperthyroidism. I recommend plant sterols and sterolins especially for patients with Graves' disease.

Moducare, which can be found at most health food stores, is one of the most popular of the plant sterol treatments.

Adults can take one capsule three times daily, or two capsules upon rising and one at bedtime. This dose may need to be increased to two to three capsules three times per day, taken one hour before meals.

Iodine

Low iodine levels are actually a leading cause of thyroid dysfunction in the world at large, although too much iodine can cause hyperthyroidism as well. Many Americans who have banned salt from their diet are beginning to experience problems. Over 70 percent of people may not be consuming enough iodine.[127] I recommend approximately 250–500 mcg of iodine a day. I commonly check iodine levels and some patients may need larger doses.

Stressed-out adrenals?

Your adrenal glands produce many different hormones, including cortisol, DHEA, pregnenolone, and testosterone. When you are under a lot of stress for a prolonged period of time, these vitally important glands can begin producing excessive cortisol. Excessive cortisol production eventually may lead to adrenal fatigue and possibly adrenal exhaustion accompanied by low cortisol production. Both of these states—excessive cortisol production and low cortisol production—can make you a poor converter of thyroxine (T4) to triiodothyronine (T3). Remember, T3 is the active form of thyroid hormone and is several times stronger than T4.

Here are some supplements that may help.

Ashwagandha

Excessive stress and high cortisol inhibits the conversion of the weaker thyroid hormone T4 to the stronger thyroid hormone T3. Ashwagandha supplements help this conversion process, and as an adaptogen, these supplements also help the adrenals.[128]

DSF or Drenamin

During extended times of stress, you can help your body balance its production of cortisol by supplementing with DSF or Drenamin. This de-stress formula is a carefully blended glandular formula that helps restore the body's adrenal function.

DHEA

DHEA is a hormone made naturally by your adrenal glands. Many call it the "youth" hormone because low levels are linked to aging. When your adrenals are exhausted, often your supply of DHEA is low, which causes hormonal regulation in your entire body to suffer. When your cortisol levels are high, DHEA levels are usually low. You can replenish this vital hormone by taking it in supplement form.

Dosage: take a small amount of DHEA. (Women usually need 10–25 mg a day; men, usually 25–50 mg a day.)

Check it out

I strongly suggest that you have all of your hormone levels checked and that you begin supplementing any hormones you are lacking. Patients with hypothyroidism and hyperthyroidism generally have low adrenal reserves and usually would benefit greatly from DHEA and DSF.

Take warning

You may be especially health conscious and currently take several supplements in order to strengthen your body. But if you have a thyroid disorder, you may need to reexamine what you're taking. Some supplements may actually aggravate your condition. Here are some supplements to watch out for.

Lipoic acid

Lipoic acid is a powerful antioxidant used by many physicians to treat diabetes, hepatitis, and psoriasis. However, lipoic acid may make you a poor converter, decreasing your ability to convert thyroxine (T4) to triiodothyronine (T3). That's the reason that some people who take lipoic acid begin exhibiting many of the symptoms of hypothyroidism.

If you have begun to take lipoic acid and have developed several symptoms of a low thyroid, you may need to either lower your dose or stop taking it altogether.

Kelp and bladder wrack

These herbs are known for having many health benefits, but they also contain lots of iodine. Too much iodine can increase your risk for developing hyperthyroidism. That's especially true if you are getting plenty of iodine in your table salt.

If you have symptoms of thyroid disorder and are taking either of these herbs, I encourage you to have your iodine level checked to make sure it is in the normal range.

Treating hypothyroidism

There are medications that can be taken to treat hypothyroidism, but if you prefer something more natural, there are options. Read below for more about both traditional medication and natural options.

Synthetic (man-made) preparations

If you have hypothyroidism, no supplement or herb can substitute for what you really need, which is thyroid hormone. Your physician probably will start you on T4, which is supplied by the major synthetic brands of T4 thyroid hormones (Synthroid, Levothroid, Levoxyl, levothyroxine, and Unithroid). Some patients, for whatever reason, don't respond as well to generic synthetic T4 hormone preparations, and so I recommend that you take the major brands mentioned above.

Synthetic T4 thyroid hormones are the standard treatment of choice for most doctors. Very rarely will a medical doctor stray from prescribing one of the four preparations listed above, or a generic version of them. Synthroid remains the top-selling thyroid hormone in the United States—its generic substitute is called *levothyroxine*.

Many patients are unable to successfully convert the T4 hormone to T3, yet their thyroid tests are normal. For these patients, I usually place them on T4 or levothyroxine and a small dose of natural thyroid extract, which contains T3. Dr. Kenneth Blanchard, an endocrinologist, has used this combination for many years with tremendous success.

Most physicians, however, only prescribe the T4 hormone, such as Synthroid. I believe that in the future, more doctors will begin to provide an appropriate mixture of T4 and T3, which is more similar to the actual hormone secretion of the thyroid gland.

A more natural path

Perhaps you've determined that you prefer to treat your hypothyroidism condition with more natural methods. Staying as close to nature as possible is often best. Nevertheless, you may imagine that only those with borderline thyroid disease have that option. But you're wrong. Natural medications exist even for those with long-term hypothyroidism. Let's take a look at some more natural options.

Natural thyroid hormone preparations, including Armour Thyroid, Biotech Thyroid, Westhroid, and Nature-throid, are medications produced from the desiccated thyroid glands of pigs. They contain both T4 and T3 hormones. Each of these natural thyroid products is essentially the same—they just have different fillers. One important note: if you have allergies to corn, take the Biotech or Nature-throid products, which have no corn fillers.

With my own patients I generally prescribe a natural thyroid hormone, such as those listed previously, in a very small amount. I use a much larger amount of T4, such as Synthroid or levothyroxine. It is usually a ratio of 95–98 percent T4 and 2–5 percent T3 as natural thyroid extract.

Again, many individuals with hypothyroidism take some form of synthetic T4, usually Synthroid, but they may not be getting all the T3 they need since many are poor converters of T4 to T3. This is the reason why they may continue to exhibit symptoms of hypothyroidism. By switching to 95–98 percent T4 and 2–5 percent T3, most symptoms of hypothyroidism can be eliminated.

Appendix A

RECOMMENDED PRODUCTS

HERBS AND SUPPLEMENTS can be purchased at your local health food store. Below are some specific products and services.

DIVINE HEALTH NUTRITIONAL PRODUCTS

1908 Boothe Circle
Longwood, FL 32750
Phone: (407) 331-7007
Website: www.drcolbert.com
E-mail: info@drcolbert.com

Divine Health Fermented Green Supremefood—a superfood blend of ten organic, fermented vegetables and four fermented grasses

Divine Health Red Supremefood—contains ten organic fruits rich in antioxidants

Diving Health Living Chia With Probiotics—organic ground chia seeds with probiotics

Divine Health Fermented Plant Protein—organic, fermented rice and pea protein with turmeric and ginger

Divine Health Fermented Beet Root Power—low in sugar and activates nitric oxide in the body

Divine Health Blood Pressure Support—contains olive leaf extract, celery seed extract, grape seed extract, and chelated magnesium

Divine Health Enhanced Multivitamin—a whole food fruit and vegetable vitamin infused with chelated minerals, active forms of the B vitamins and methyltetrahydrofolate (MTHF)

Divine Health Brain Defense—contains curcumin, pomegranate and pterostilbene to defend the brain from oxidative stress

Divine Health Living Serene-3—an adaptogenic formula for stress that includes ginseng (GS15-4) that has fifteen times increased absorption, ashwaghanda and Rhodiola

Divine Health Prostate Formula—contains beta-sitosterol, Boswellia, lycopene, pumpkin seed, saw palmetto, selenium, and zinc

OTHER SUPPLEMENTS PROVIDED BY DR. COLBERT'S OFFICE

Phone: (407) 331-7007

Most supplements in this manual can be found in health food stores. There are special supplements that are difficult to find.

Coromega Omega-3—absorbed 300 percent more effectively than fish oil soft gels, extremely high purity, very low in lipid peroxides, has a great taste

Mastic Gum and DGL—contains both supplements for reflux

Neuro-Mag Powder—contains magnesium L-threonate, calcium, and vitamin D_3

Mucuna—contains 60 percent L-Dopa in a 100 mg capsule

Vascuzyme—contains proteolytic enzymes

Krill oil with astaxanthin

Hyaluronic Acid low molecular weight

RiboCeine (MaxOne or Cellgevity)

Curcumin

De-Stress Formula (DSF)—adrenal rebuilder formula

ALA Max—alpha lipoic acid, 600 mg

Gamma E—mixed tocopherols and tocotrienols

Crila—an herb from Vietnam that supports the prostate

Stress Relief Drops—mineral drops for stress

Sinus Formula—support for environmental allergies and hay fever

INSTITUTE FOR BETTER BONE HEALTH (IBBH) BONE AND JOINT SUPPLEMENTS

1908 Boothe Circle
Longwood, FL 32750
info@bonehealthnow.com
kyle@bonehealthnow.com
1-800-242-6149

IBBH Silical 1—contains calcium, magnesium, and vitamin D_3

IBBH Silical 2—contains silicon, vitamin K_2, boron, vitamin C, inositol, and L-arginine for bone support

IBBH Joint Formula—contains UCII collagen, ASU to support collagen production, and Boswellia to decrease inflammation

Bioidentical Hormone Replacement Therapy (BHRT) and Anti-Aging Medicine

Access directory of physicians at the American Academy of Anti-Aging Medicine.

Website: www.worldhealth.net

Cell Science Systems

852 S. Military Trail
Deerfield Beach, FL 33442
800-875-5228
Website: www.alcat.com
E-mail: info@alcat.com
Food Sensitivity Testing: ALCAT

Appendix B

FODMAP DIET

ON THE FODMAP (fermentable oligosaccharides, disaccharides, monosaccharides, and polyols) diet, avoid fruits with fructose, stone fruits, high-fructose corn syrup, dairy, wheat, onion, garlic, beans, and lentils. Eat foods such as beef, chicken, almond milk, small amounts of cream cheese or hard cheeses, bananas, berries, leafy greens, potatoes, tomatoes, and more. Follow this diet for six weeks before adding foods in one at a time. This will help you identify any foods that are triggers.[1]

NOTES

Chapter 1: Your Nutritional Deficit

1. Robert H. Fletcher and Kathleen M. Fairfield, "Vitamins for Chronic Disease Prevention in Adults," *Journal of the American Medical Association* 287 (2002): 3127–3129.

2. Ibid.

3. Joseph Mercola, "11 Most Common Nutrient Deficiencies," Mercola.com, October 19, 2015, accessed June 20, 2016, http://articles.mercola.com/sites/articles/archive/2015/10/19/most-common-nutrient-deficiencies.aspx.

4. "Why You Can't Eat Well," The Results Project, referenced in Don Colbert, "Curbing the Toxic Onslaught," *NutriNews*, August 2005, accessed August 15, 2016, https://www.douglaslabs.ca/pdf/nutrinews/Detoxification%20III.pdf.

5. Rex Beach, "Modern Miracle Men," S. Doc. No. 264 (1936), accessed August 15, 2016, http://www.senate.gov/reference/resources/pdf/modernmiraclemen.pdf.

6. "Vegetables Without Vitamins," *Life Extension*, March 2001, accessed August 15, 2016, http://www.lifeextension.com/magazine/2001/3/report_vegetables/page-01.

7. "Acid Rain Threatens Future Productivity of Forests, Research Shows," ScienceDaily, March 15, 1999, accessed August 15, 2016, https://www.sciencedaily.com/releases/1999/03/990315081321.htm.

8. "Dirt Poor: Have Fruits and Vegetables Become Less Nutritious?", EarthTalk, editors Roddy Scheer and Doug Moss, *Scientific American*, April 27, 2011, accessed August 15, 2016, http://www.scientificamerican.com/article/soil-depletion-and-nutrition-loss/.

9. "The World's Healthiest Foods," The George Mateljan Foundation, accessed October 16, 2015, http://www.whfoods.org/foodstoc.php.

10. "Digestive Disorders," LifeExtension.org, accessed August 15, 2016, http://www.lef.org/protocols/prtcl-044.shtml.

Chapter 2: What's in Your Food and Water

1. "How We Eat," *Rural Migration News*, 2, no. 4 (October 1996), accessed August 15, 2016, https://migration.ucdavis.edu/rmn/more.php?id=158.

2. "Life Expectancy," Centers for Disease Control and Prevention, accessed August 15, 2016, http://www.cdc.gov/nchs/fastats/life-expectancy.htm; "High Blood Pressure Facts," Centers for Disease Control and Prevention, accessed August 15, 2016, http://www.cdc.gov/bloodpressure/facts.htm; "Adult Obesity Facts," Centers for Disease Control and Prevention, accessed August 15, 2016, http://www.cdc.gov/obesity/data/adult.html.

3. Sue Hughes, "Alzheimer's Cases May Triple by 2050," WebMD, February 7, 2013, accessed July 21, 2016, http://www.webmd.com/alzheimers/news/20130207/alzheimers-cases-may-triple.

4. Elizabeth Renter, "Researchers Link MSG to Weight Gain, Obesity," Natural Society, February 24, 2013, accessed July 21, 2016, http://naturalsociety.com/flavor-enhancer-msg-linked-to-weight-gain/.

5. Daniel J. DeNoon, "Drink More Diet Soda, Gain More Weight?" WebMD, June 13, 2005, accessed June 20, 2016, http://www.webmd.com/diet/20050613/drink-more-diet-soda-gain-more-weight?printing=true.

6. Eric Schlosser, *Fast Food Nation* (New York: Houghton Mifflin, 2001).

7. Michelle Jamrikso, "Americans' Spending on Dining Out Just Overtook Grocery Sales for the First Time Ever," *Bloomberg*, April 14, 2015, accessed June 20, 2016, http://www.bloomberg.com/news/articles/2015-04-14/americans-spending-on-dining-out-just-overtook-grocery-sales-for-the-first-time-ever.

8. "Meat Drippings (Lard, Meat Tallow, Mutton Tallow)," CalorieKing.com, accessed June 20, 2016, http://tinyurl.com/jku32an.

9. "Know Your Fats," American Heart Association, updated March 18, 2016, accessed June, 2016, http://www.heart.org/HEARTORG/Conditions/Cholesterol/PreventionTreatmentofHighCholesterol/Know-Your-Fats_UCM_305628_Article.jsp#.ViJr8it1z3U.

10. Dina Spector, "Here's How Many Days a Person Can Survive Without Water," Business Insider, May 9, 2014, accessed August 15, 2016, http://www.businessinsider.com/how-many-days-can-you-survive-without-water-2014-5.

11. Barbara Levine, "Hydration 101: The Case for Drinking Enough Water," HealthPointe 2.0, accessed August 15, 2016, http://www.myhealthpointe.com/health_Nutrition_news/index.cfm?Health=10.

12. D. A. Mansfield, "What Percentage of the Human Body Is Water, and How Is This Determined?" *Boston Globe*, January 12, 1998, accessed August 15, 2016, https://www.highbeam.com/doc/1P2-8457255.html.

CHAPTER 3: UNEXPECTED SOURCES OF TOXINS

1. "Cancer Facts & Figures 2015," American Cancer Society, accessed August 16, 2016, http://www.cancer.org/acs/groups/content/@editorial/documents/document/acspc-044552.pdf.

2. "Tobacco Related Cancer Fact Sheet," American Cancer Society, updated February 21, 2014, accessed June 20, 2016, http://www.cancer.org/cancer/cancercauses/tobaccocancer/tobacco-related-cancer-fact-sheet; Harvard Reports on Cancer Prevention, "Volume I: Human Causes of Cancer," *Cancer Causes and Control* 7 (Supplement, November 1996).

3. Gene Marine and Judith Van Allen, *Food Pollution—the Violation of Our Inner Ecology* (Canada: Holt, Rinehart, and Winston, 1972), referenced in Judy Campbell et al., "Nutritional Characteristics of Organic, Freshly Stone-Ground, Sourdough and Conventional Breads," Ecological Agricultural Projects, accessed November 16, 2015, referenced in Colbert, "Curbing the Toxic Onslaught."

4. "PCBs and DDT: Banned but Still With Us," Pollution in People, July 2006, accessed October 19, 2015, http://www.pollutioninpeople.org/toxics/pcbs_ddt.

5. T. S. Johnson, "Diagnosis and Treatment of Five Parasites: Enterobus vermicularis, Giardia lamblia, Trichuris trichuira, Ascaris lumbricoides, Entamoeba histolytica," *Drug Intelligence and Clinical Pharmacy* 15, no. 2 (1981): 103–110.

6. Michael D. Gershon, *The Second Brain* (New York: HarperPerennial, 1999), 152–153.

7. Don Colbert, *What You Don't Know May Be Killing You* (Lake Mary, FL: Siloam, 2004); also, Don Colbert, *Get Healthy Through Detox and Fasting* (Lake Mary, FL: Siloam, 2006).

8. Greg Ciola, "Mercury: The Unsuspected Killer!" *Crusader Special Report*, April/May 2004, 3, referenced in Colbert, "Curbing the Toxic Onslaught."

9. Donald W. Miller Jr., "Mercury on the Mind," LewRockwell.com, accessed August 16, 2016, https://www.lewrockwell.com/2004/09/donald-w-miller-jr-md/the-curse-of-mercury-in-vaccines/, referenced in Colbert, "Curbing the Toxic Onslaught."

10. Walter J. Crinnion, "Environmental Medicine, Part Three: Long-Term Effects of Chronic Low-Dose Mercury Exposure," *Alternative Medicine Review* 5, no. 3 (2000): 209–223, accessed June 21, 2016, http://www.altmedrev.com/publications/5/3/209.pdf.

11. Agency for Toxic Substances and Disease Registry, "A Toxicology Curriculum for Communities Trainer's Manual," lecture notes for module four, accessed June 21, 2016, http://www.atsdr.cdc.gov/training/toxmanual/modules/4/lecturenotes.html.

12. "Safe Substitutes at Home: Non-toxic Household Products," Fact Sheet, http://infohouse.p2ric.org/ref/07/06634.pdf, accessed June 21, 2016, excerpted from Gary A. Davis and Em Turner, "Safe Substitutes at Home: Non-toxic Household Products," working paper, University of Tennessee—Knoxville Waste Management Institute.

13. Ibid.

14. Ibid.

15. Environmental Working Group, "Ethyl Benzene," accessed June 21, 2016, http://www.ewg.org/sites/bodyburden1/popup_chemdetail.php?chem_id=90001&sub=s4.

16. Christian Nordqvist, *Medical News Today*, "High Benzene Levels Found in Some Soft Drinks," May 20, 2006, accessed June 21, 2016, http://www.medicalnewstoday.com/articles/43763.php.

17. "Case Studies in Environmental Medicine: Tetrachloroethylene Toxicity," Agency for Toxic Substances and Disease Registry, May 2008, accessed June 22, 2016, http://www.atsdr.cdc.gov/csem/pce/docs/pce.pdf.

18. N. Hanioka et al., "Interaction of 2,4,4'-trichloro-2'-hydroxydiphenyl Ether With Microsomal Cytochrome P450-dependent Monooxygenases in Rat Liver," *Chemosphere* 33, no. 2 (July 1996): 265–276; H. N. Bhargava and P. A. Leonard, "Triclosan: Applications and Safety," *American Journal of Infection Control* 24, no. 3 (June 1996): 209–218.

19. Garth H. Rauscher, David Shore, and Dale P. Sandler, "Hair Dye Use and Risk of Adult Acute Leukemia," *American Journal of Epidemiology* 160, no. 1 (2004): 19–25.

Chapter 4: How Stress Depletes Your Body

1. John Hagee, *The Seven Secrets* (Lake Mary, FL: Charisma House, 2004), 31.

2. Tara Parker-Pope, "Health Journal: Secrets of Successful Aging," *Wall Street Journal*, June 20, 2005, R-3.

3. D. A. Snowdon et al., "Linguistic Ability in Early Life and Cognitive Function and Alzheimer's Disease in Late Life. Findings From the Nun Study," *Journal of the American Medical Association* 275 (February 21, 1996): 528–532.

4. S. Kennedy, J. K. Kiecolt-Glaser, and R. Glaser, "Immunological Consequences of Acute and Chronic Stressors: Mediating Role of Interpersonal Stressors," *British Journal of Medical Psychology* 61 (1988): 77–85.

5. H. J. Eysenck et al., "Personality Type, Smoking Habit, and Their Interaction as Predictors of Cancer and Coronary Disease," *Personality and Individual Difference* 9, no. 2 (1988): 479–495.

6. Ibid.

7. Ibid.

8. D. Wayne, "Reactions to Stress," found in Identifying Stress, a series offered by the Health-Net & Stress Management web site, February 1998.

9. P. M. Plotsky et al., "PsychoNeural Endocrinology of Depression: Hypothalamic-Pituitary-Adrenal Axis," *Psychoneurology* 21, no. 2 (1998): 293–306.

10. "Stress in America Findings," American Psychological Association, accessed October 13, 2016, https://www.apa.org/news/press/releases/stress/2010/national-report.pdf.

11. Don Colbert, *Stress Less* (Lake Mary, FL: Siloam, 2005).

12. Doc Childre and Howard Martin, *The HeartMath Solution* (San Francisco: HarperSanFrancisco, 2000).

13. David L. Rambo, "Come Apart Before You Fall Apart," March 1993, in Swenson, *The Overload Syndrome*, 181.

CHAPTER 5: YOUR WEIGHT AND METABOLISM

1. Barbara Bushman and Janice Clark-Young, *Action Plan for Menopause* (Champaign, IL: American College of Sports Medicine, 2005), 68–70.

2. Ibid.

3. *Webster's New World College Dictionary*, fourth edition (Foster City, CA: IDG Books Worldwide Inc., 2001), s.v. "metabolism."

4. Jim Harvey, "Measuring BMR in the Pulmonary Lab," *FOCUS: Journal for Respiratory Care and Sleep Medicine* (July 1, 2006), accessed June 24, 2016, http://www.thefreelibrary.com/Measuring+BMR+in+the+Pulmonary+lab.-a0186218061.

5. Osama Hamdy, "Obesity," eMedicine.com, May 21, 2009, accessed June 24, 2016, http://emedicine.medscape.com/article/123702-overview.

6. James Levine et al., "Interindividual Variation in Posture Allocation: Possible Role in Human Obesity," *Science* 307, no. 5709 (2005): 584–586.

7. Lawrence C. Wood, David S. Cooper, and E. Chester Ridgway, *Your Thyroid: A Home Reference* (New York: Ballantine Books, 1995).

8. Karilee Halo Shames et al., "The Thyroid Dance: Nursing Approaches to Autoimmune Low Thyroid," *AWHONN Lifelines* 6, no. 1 (2002): 52–59.

Chapter 6: An Alphabet of Nutrition: Vitamins A, C, D, E, K

1. Alanna Moshfegh, Joseph Goodman, and Linda Cleveland, "What We Eat in America, NHANES 2001–2002: Usual Nutrient Intakes From Food Compared to Dietary Reference Intakes," US Department of Agriculture, Agricultural Research Service, 2005, accessed June 24, 2016, http://www.ars.usda.gov/SP2UserFiles/Place/80400530/pdf/0102/usualintaketables2001-02.pdf.

2. Phyllis A. Balch, *Prescription for Nutritional Healing*, rev. and expanded edition (New York: Avery Books, 2000), 14–15.

3. "Vitamin A: Fact Sheet for Health Professionals," National Institutes of Health Office of Dietary Supplements, NIH Clinical Center, accessed June 24, 2016, https://ods.od.nih.gov/factsheets/VitaminA-HealthProfessional/#h2.

4. Ibid.

5. K. J. Rothman, L. L. Moore, and M. R. Singer, "Tertogenecity of High Vitamin A Intake," *New England Journal of Medicine* 333 (1995): 1369–1373.

6. Joseph E. Pizzorno Jr. and Michael T. Murray, eds., *Textbook of Natural Medicine* (New York: Churchill Livingston, 1999), 1013.

7. From an e-mail from Cathy Leet, BSN, Director of Market Development, Integrative Therapeutics Inc., to author's office, Tuesday, January 31, 2006.

8. "Dietary Supplement Fact Sheet: Vitamin A and Carotenoids," National Institutes of Health Office of Dietary Supplements, NIH Clinical Center, accessed September 9, 2008, http://ods.od.nih.gov/factsheets/vitamina.asp; Dana Angelo White, "Nutrient to Know: Vitamin A," Food Network, June 11, 2009, accessed August 23, 2016, http://blog.foodnetwork.com/healthyeats/2009/06/11/nutrient-to-know-vitamin-a/; Betty Kovacs, "Vitamin and Calcium Supplements," MedicineNet.com, Accessed August 23, 2016, http://www.medicinenet.com/vitamins_and_calcium_supplements/page6.htm; "Vitamin A: Fact Sheet for Health Professionals," National Institutes of Health Office of Dietary Supplements.

9. Pizzorno and Murray, *Textbook of Natural Medicine*, 1007–1013.

10. Ross Bloom, "92% of U.S. Population Have Vitamin Deficiency. Are You One of Them?" TheBiostation.com, February 3, 2014, accessed August 17, 2016, http://thebiostation.com/resource-center/wellness/92-of-u-s-population-have-vitamin-deficiency-are-you-one-of-them/.

11. Moshfegh, Goodman, and Cleveland "What We Eat in America, NHANES 2001–2002: Usual Nutrient Intakes From Food Compared to Dietary Reference Intakes."

12. "Extension Fact Sheet: Vitamin C (Ascorbic Acid)," Ohio State University, accessed June 24, 2016, http://ohioline.osu.edu/factsheet/HYG-5552.

13. "Symptoms of Vitamin C deficiency," RightDiagnosis.com, accessed August 17, 2016, http://www.rightdiagnosis.com/v/vitamin_c_deficiency/symptoms.htm.

14. Pizzorno and Murray, *Textbook of Natural Medicine*, 549, 836, 915–916.

15. Bloom, "92% of U.S. Population Have Vitamin Deficiency. Are You One of Them?"

16. Balch, *Prescription for Nutritional Healing*, 21.

17. "Dietary Supplement Fact Sheet: Vitamin D," National Institutes of Health Office of Dietary Supplements, NIH Clinical Center, accessed October 24, 2015, https://ods.od.nih.gov/factsheets/VitaminD-HealthProfessional/.

18. According to an analysis published in 2004 and based on the Third National Health and Nutrition Examination Survey (NHANES III).

19. Raloff, "Understanding Vitamin D Deficiency."

20. "Dietary Supplement Fact Sheet: Vitamin D," National Institutes of Health Office of Dietary Supplements.

21. Ibid.

22. "Sources of Calcium," National Osteoporosis Foundation, accessed August 19, 2016, https://www.nof.org/patients/treatment/calciumvitamin-d/.

23. "Vitamin D Deficiency May Increase Risk of Hip Fracture in Older Women," National Institute on Aging, April 27, 1999, accessed August 19, 2016, https://www.nia.nih.gov/newsroom/1999/04/vitamin-d-deficiency-may-increase-risk-hip-fracture-older-women.

24. Moshfegh, Goodman, and Cleveland, "What We Eat in America, NHANES 2001–2002: Usual Nutrient Intakes From Food Compared to Dietary Reference Intakes."

25. "Is Vitamin E Beneficial or Harmful?," Nutrition Advisor, accessed August 22, 2016, http://www.nutritionadvisor.com/vitamin-E.php.

26. "Vitamin E," National Institutes of Health Office of Dietary Supplements, NIH Clinical Center, accessed August 22, 2016, https://ods.od.nih.gov/factsheets/VitaminE-HealthProfessional/.

27. Eva Lonn et al., "Effects of Long-Term Vitamin E Supplementation on Cardiovascular Events and Cancer," *Journal of the American Medical Association* 293, no. 11 (March 16, 2005): 1338–1347.

28. "The Effect of Vitamin E and Beta Carotene on the Incidence of Lung Cancer and Other Cancers in Male Smokers," *New England Journal of Medicine* 330, no. 15 (April 14, 1994), accessed August 22, 2016, http://atbcstudy.cancer.gov/pdfs/atbc33010291994.pdf.

29. K. J. Helzlsouer et. al., "Association Between Alpha-Tocopherol, Gamma-Tocopherol, Selenium, and Subsequent Prostate Cancer," *Journal of the National Cancer Institute* 92, no. 24 (December 2000): 1966–1967.

30. Moshfegh, Goodman, and Cleveland, "What We Eat in America, NHANES 2001–2002: Usual Nutrient Intakes From Food Compared to Dietary Reference Intakes."

31. Balch, *Prescription for Nutritional Healing*, 22–23; "Vitamin K," Linus Pauling Institute Micronutrient Information Center, Oregon State University, accessed August 19, 2016, http://lpi.oregonstate.edu/infocenter/vitamins/vitaminK/index.html.

32. "Vitamin K: Fact Sheet for Health Professionals," National Institutes of Health, Office of Dietary Supplements, updated February 11, 2016, accessed August 22, 2016, https://ods.od.nih.gov/factsheets/VitaminK-HealthProfessional/.

33. Ibid.

34. Balch, *Prescription for Nutritional Healing*, 23.

35. Y. Seyama and H. Wachi, "Atherosclerosis and Matrix Dystrophy," *Journal of Atherosclerosis and Thrombosis* 11, no. 5 (2004): 236–245.

36. A. M. Stapleton and R. L. Rydall, "Crystal Matrix Protein—Getting Blood Out of a Stone," *Mineral and Electrolyte Metabolism* 20, no. 6 (1994): 399–409.

37. William Davis, "Protecting Bone and Arterial Health With Vitamin K_2," *Life Extension Magazine*, March 2008, accessed July 25, 2016, http://www.lifeextension.com/magazine/2008/3/protecting-bone-and-arterial-health-with-vitamin-k2/Page-01.

Chapter 7: The B Vitamins: Nutrition's First Family

1. "Thiamin: Fact Sheet for Health Professionals," National Institutes of Health, updated February 11, 2016, accessed July 22, 2016, https://ods.od.nih.gov/factsheets/Thiamin-HealthProfessional/; "Thiamin: Fact Sheet for Consumers," National Institutes of Health, updated April 13, 2016, accessed July 22, 2016, https://ods.od.nih.gov/factsheets/Thiamin-Consumer/; "Health Benefits of Vitamin B_1 or Thiamine," Organic Facts, accessed July 22, 2016, https://www.organicfacts.net/health-benefits/vitamins/vitamin-b1-or-thiamine.html.

2. "Riboflavin: Fact Sheet for Health Professionals," National Institutes of Health, updated February 11, 2016, accessed July 22, 2016, https://ods.od.nih.gov/factsheets/Riboflavin-HealthProfessional/; "Riboflavin: Fact Sheet for Consumers," National Institutes of Health, updated February 17, 2016, accessed July 22, 2016, https://ods.od.nih.gov/factsheets/Riboflavin-consumer/.

3. "Niacin (Vitamin B_3)," WebMD, reviewed May 1, 2015, accessed July 22, 2016, http://www.webmd.com/diet/supplement-guide-niacin?page=1.

4. A. Fidanz, "Therapeutic Action of Pantothenic Acid," *International Journal for Vitamin and Nutrition Research* 24, supplement (1983): 53–67.

5. Alfred H. Merrill Jr. and J. Michael Henderson, "Diseases Associated With Defects in Vitamin B_6 Metabolism or Utilization," *Annual Review of Nutrition* 7 (July 1987): 135–156.

6. Moshfegh, Goodman, and Cleveland, "What We Eat in America, NHANES 2001–2002: Usual Nutrient Intakes From Food Compared to Dietary Reference Intakes," U.S. Department of Agriculture, Agricultural Research Service, accessed October 24, 2015, http://www.ars.usda.gov/SP2UserFiles/Place/80400530/pdf/0102/usualintaketables2001-02.pdf.

7. J. E. Leklem, "Vitamin B_6," in M. E. Shils et al., ed., *Modern Nutrition in Health and Disease*, 9th ed. (Baltimore: Williams and Wilkins, 1999), 413–421.

8. "Vitamin B_6: Dietary Supplement Fact Sheet," National Institutes of Health, updated February 11, 2016, accessed July 22, 2016, https://ods.od.nih.gov/factsheets/VitaminB6-HealthProfessional/; "Vitamin B6—Pyridoxine," Whfoods.org, accessed July 22, 2016, http://www.whfoods.com/genpage.php?tname=nutrient&dbid=108#foodsources.

9. "Homocysteine," Wiley.com, accessed August 30, 2016, http://www.wiley.com/college/boyer/0470003790/cutting_edge/homocysteine/homocysteine.htm.

10. "Biotin," WebMD, accessed July 22, 2016, http://www.webmd.com/vitamins-and-supplements/supplement-guide-biotin.

11. "Vitamin B_9 (Folic Acid)," University of Maryland Medical Center, reviewed August 5, 2015, accessed July 22, 2016, http://umm.edu/health/medical/altmed/supplement/vitamin-b9-folic-acid; "Folate: Dietary Supplement Fact Sheet," National

Institutes of Health, updated April 20, 2016, accessed July 22, 2016, https://ods.od.nih.gov/factsheets/Folate-HealthProfessional/.

12. R. M. Russell, "A Minimum of 13,500 Deaths Annual From Coronary Artery Disease Could Be Prevented by Increasing Folate Intake to Reduce Homocysteine Levels," *Journal of the American Medical Association* 275 (1996): 1828–1829.

13. M. Fava et al., "Folate, Vitamin B_{12}, and Homocysteine in Major Depressive Disorder," *American Journal of Psychiatry* 153, no. 2 (1997): 426–428.

14. Dr. Mercola, "11 Most Common Nutrient Deficiencies," Mercola, October 19, 2015, accessed July 22, 2016, http://articles.mercola.com/sites/articles/archive/2015/10/19/most-common-nutrient-deficiencies.aspx.

15. Ralph Carmel, "Subtle Cobalamin Deficiency," *Annals of Internal Medicine* 124, no. 3 (February 1, 1996): 338–340.

16. "Getting Enough B_{12}?," Tufts University, E-News, September 10, 2001, accessed August 22, 2016, http://enews.tufts.edu/stories/1263/2001/09/10/GettingEnoughB12/.

17. S. P. Stabler, J. Lindenbaum, and R. H. Allen, "Vitamin B_{12} Deficiency in the Elderly: Current Dilemmas," *American Journal of Clinical Nutrition* 66 (October 1997): 741–749.

CHAPTER 8: DIGGING FOR GOLD: MINERALS AND YOUR BODY

1. Dana E. King et al., "Dietary Magnesium and C-Reactive Protein Levels," *Journal of American College of Nutrition* 24, no. 3 (June 2005): 166–171.

2. National Institutes of Health Office of Dietary Supplements, "Dietary Supplement Fact Sheet: Magnesium," NIH Clinical Center, updated February 11, 2016, accessed July 22, 2016, https://ods.od.nih.gov/factsheets/Magnesium-HealthProfessional/.

3. National Institutes of Health Office of Dietary Supplements, "Dietary Supplement Fact Sheet: Calcium," NIH Clinical Center, updated June 1, 2016, accessed June 29, 2016, https://ods.od.nih.gov/factsheets/Calcium-HealthProfessional/.

4. Ibid.

5. Ibid.

6. Ibid.

7. "Important News on Osteoporosis and Bone Health," CalciumInfo.com, accessed August 30, 2016, https://web.archive.org/web/20060302040120/http://calciuminfo.com/; "Calcium Deficiency," MDHealth.com, accessed August 30, 2016, http://www.md-health.com/Calcium-Deficiency.html.

8. Rekha Mankad, "Heart Attack," February 11, 2016, accessed July 22, 2016, http://www.mayoclinic.org/diseases-conditions/heart-attack/expert-answers/calcium-supplements/faq-20058352.

9. Adam Drewnowski, Matthieu Malliot, and Colin Rehm, "Reducing the Sodium-Potassium Ratio in the US Diet: A Challenge for Public Health," *The American Journal of Clinical Nutrition* 96, no. 2 (August 1, 2012), accessed June 28, 2016, http://ajcn.nutrition.org/content/96/2/439.full.pdf+html.

10. "Potassium," WebMD, reviewed March 1, 2015, accessed July 22, 2016, http://www.webmd.com/diet/supplement-guide-potassium; "The American Heart Association's Diet and Lifestyle Recommendations," American Heart Association, updated

January 20, 2016, July 22, 2016, http://www.heart.org/HEARTORG/HealthyLiving/Diet-and-Lifestyle-Recommendations_UCM_305855_Article.jsp#.V5J0JbgrLcs.

11. Moshfegh, Goodman, and Cleveland, "What We Eat in America, NHANES 2001–2002."

12. "Dietary Guidelines for Americans: 2015–2020," USDA, December 2015, accessed July 22, 2016, https://health.gov/dietaryguidelines/2015/resources/2015-2020_Dietary_Guidelines.pdf.

13. Joseph G. Hollowell et al., "Iodine Nutrition in the United States. Trends and Public Health Implications: Iodine Excretion Data from National Health and Nutrition Examination Surveys I and III (1971–1974 and 1988–1994)," *Journal of Clinical Endocrinology &* http://jcem.endojournals.org/cgi/content/full/83/10/3401 *Metabolism* 83, no. 10 (October 1998): 3401–3408, accessed June 28, 2016, http://jcem.endojournals.org/cgi/content/full/83/10/3401.

14. MedNews.am, "Why are women more likely to have thyroid disease than men?" accessed November 5, 2015, http://med.news.am/eng/news/1155/why-are-women-more-likely-to-have-thyroid-disease-than-men.html.

15. "Dietary Guidelines for Americans: 2015–2020," USDA.

16. "Food Sources of Vitamins and Minerals," WebMD, reviewed October 6, 2014, accessed July 22, 2016, http://www.webmd.com/food-recipes/vitamin-mineral-sources?page=1.

17. "Vitamins and Minerals: How Much Should You Take?" WebMD, reviewed June 23, 2016, accessed July 22, 2016, http://www.webmd.com/vitamins-and-supplements/vitamins-minerals-how-much-should-you-take?page=3.

18. "Chloride in Diet," Medline Plus, updated February 2, 2015, accessed July 22, 2016, https://medlineplus.gov/ency/article/002417.htm.

19. "Dietary Guidelines for Americans: 2015–2020," USDA.

20. "Iron Dietary Supplement Fact Sheet," National Institutes of Health, accessed October 13, 2016, https://ods.od.nih.gov/factsheets/Iron-HealthProfessional/.

21. "Dietary Guidelines for Americans: 2015–2020," USDA.

22. Ibid.

23. "Chromium: Dietary Supplement Fact Sheet," National Institutes of Health, updated November 4, 2013, accessed July 22, 2016, https://ods.od.nih.gov/factsheets/Chromium-HealthProfessional/.

24. "Dietary Guidelines for Americans: 2015–2020," USDA.

25. "Vitamins and Minerals: How Much Should You Take?," WebMD, reviewed June 23, 2016, accessed July 22, 2016, http://www.webmd.com/vitamins-and-supplements/vitamins-minerals-how-much-should-you-take?page=3.

26. "Boron," *MedlinePlus*, National Institutes of Health, accessed October 13, 2016, https://medlineplus.gov/druginfo/natural/894.html.

Chapter 9: Your Need for Antioxidants

1. P. Mecocci et al., "Plasma Antioxidants and Longevity: a Study on Healthy Centenarians," *Free Radical Biology and Medicine* 28, no. 8 (September 2000): 1243–1248.

2. V. P. Chernyshov et al., "Effects of Rec. Comp. on Immune System on Chernobyl Children With RRD," *International Journal of Immunorehabilitation* 5 (May 1997): 72.

3. Sally K. Nelson et al., "The Induction of Human Superoxide Dismutase and Catalase in Vivo: A Fundamentally New Approach to Antioxidant Therapy," *Free Radical Biology and Medicine* 40 (2006): 341–347.

4. Lester Packer, *The Antioxidant Miracle* (New York: John Wiley and Sons, Inc., 1999).

5. "Lipoic Acid," Linus Pauling Institute Micronutrient Information Center, Oregon State University, accessed June 29, 2016, http://lpi.oregonstate.edu/mic/dietary-factors/lipoic-acid.

6. C. W. Shults et al., "Effects of Coenzyme Q_{10} in Early Parkinson Disease," *Archives of Neurology* 59 (2002): 1541–1550; "A Randomized, Placebo-Controlled Trial of Coenzyme Q_{10} and Remacemide in Huntington's Disease," The Huntington Study Group, *Neurology* 57 (2001): 397–404; P. Langsjoen et al., "The Aging Heart: Reversal of Diastolic Dysfunction Through the Use of Oral CoQ_{10} in the Elderly," in *Anti-Aging Medical Therapeutics*, R. M. Klatz and R. Goldman, eds. (n.p.: Health Quest Publications, 1997), 113–120; C. W. Shults, "Absorption, Tolerability, and Effects on Mitochondrial Activity of Oral Coenzyme Q_{10} in Parkinsonian Patients," *Neurology* 50 (1998): 793–795; K. Folkers, "Lovastatin Decreases Coenzyme Q Levels in Humans," *Proceedings of the National Academy of the Sciences of the United States of America* 87, no. 22 (1990): 8931–8934; C. W. Shults et al., "Pilot Trial of High Dosages of Coenzyme Q_{10} in Patients With Parkinson's Disease," *Experimental Neurology* 188, no. 2 (August 2004): 491–494.

7. Perry Marcone, "Generate Fresh Mitochondria With PQQ," *Life Extension Magazine*, February 2011, accessed July 25, 2016, http://www.lifeextension.com/magazine/2011/2/Generate-Fresh-Mitochondria-with-PQQ/Page-01.

CHAPTER 10: PHYTONUTRIENTS: THE RAINBOW OF HEALTH

1. George Mateljan Foundation, "What Is the Special Nutritional Power Found in Fruits and Vegetables?" accessed August 23, 2016, http://www.whfoods.com/genpage.php?tname=faq&dbid=4.

2. Balch, *Prescription for Nutritional Healing*, 9.

3. "Amazon Expedition: Threats and Solutions," Greenpeace, accessed June 30, 2016, http://www.greenpeace.org/international/Global/international/planet-2/report/2001/9/amazon-threats-and-solutions.pdf.

4. Latetia V. Moore and Frances E. Thompson, "Adults Meeting Fruit and Vegetable Intake Recommendations—United States, 2013," Centers for Disease Control and Prevention, July 10, 2015, accessed August 23, 2016, http://www.cdc.gov/mmwr/preview/mmwrhtml/mm6426a1.htm.

5. E. Giovannucci et al., "Intake of Carotenoids and Retinol in Relation to Risk of Prostate Cancer," *Journal of the National Cancer Institute* 87 (December 6, 1995): 1767–1776.

6. "Prostate Cancer Risk Factors," WebMD.com, accessed August 23, 2016, www.webmd.com/prostate-cancer/guide/prostate-cancer-risk-factors.

7. Ethan Trex, "Are Tomatoes Fruits or Vegetables?" MentalFloss.com, June 9, 2010, accessed June 30, 2016, http://mentalfloss.com/article/24881/are-tomatoes-fruits-or-vegetables; *Nix v. Hedden*, No. 137, May 10, 1893, accessed June 30, 2016, http://caselaw.findlaw.com/us-supreme-court/149/304.html.

8. "The Effect of Vitamin E and Beta-Carotene on the Incidence of Lung Cancer and Other Cancers in Male Smokers," *New England Journal of Medicine* 330, no. 15 (April 14, 1994): 1029–1035.

9. J. Michael Gaziano et al., "A Prospective Study of Consumption of Carotenoids in Fruits and Vegetables and Decreased Cardiovascular Mortality in the Elderly," *Annals of Epidemiology* 5, no. 4 (July 1995): 255–260.

10. J. M. Seddon et al., "Dietary Carotenoids, Vitamins A, C, and E, and Advanced Age-Related Macular Degeneration," *Journal of the American Medical Association* 272 (1994): 1413–1420.

11. B. B. Aggarwal and H. Ichikawa, "Molecular Targets and Anticancer Potential of Indole-3-Carbinol and Its Derivatives," *Cell Cycle* 4, no. 9 (September 2004): 1201–1215.

12. H. Lucille, "Assessing the Underlying Cause," in *Creating and Maintaining Balance: A Woman's Guide to Safe, Natural, Hormone Health* (Boulder, CO: IMPAKT Health, 2004), 15–25.

13. John C. Martin, "Can Curcumin Prevent Alzheimer's Disease?," *Life Extension Magazine*, December 2004, accessed July 1, 2016, http://www.lifeextension.com/Magazine/2004/12/report_curcumin/Page-01.

14. I. Alwi et al., "The Effect of Curcumin on Lipid Levels in Patients With Acute Coronary Syndrome," October 4, 2008, accessed July 1, 2016, http://www.ncbi.nlm.nih.gov/pubmed/19151449.

15. Judy McBride, "High-ORAC Foods May Slow Aging," United States Department of Agriculture, Agricultural Research Service, February 8, 1999, accessed July 1, 2016, http://www.ars.usda.gov/is/pr/1999/990208.htm.

16. Ronald L. Prior et al., "Can Foods Forestall Aging?" *AgResearch Magazine*, February 1999, accessed July 1, 2016, http://www.ars.usda.gov/is/AR/archive/feb99/aging0299.htm?pf=1.

17. X. Wu et al., "Lipophilic and Hydrophilic Antioxidant Capacities of Common Foods in the United States," *Journal of Agricultural and Food Chemistry* 52, no. 12 (June 16, 2004): 4026–4037.

18. Tiesha D. Johnson, "All About Supplements: Blueberries," *Life Extension*, September 2006, 88.

19. Ibid.

Chapter 11: The Importance of Healthy Fats

1. "Nutrition Calculator," McDonald's, accessed August 23, 2016, https://www.mcdonalds.com/us/en-us/about-our-food/nutrition-calculator.html.

2. W. C. Willet et al., "Intake of Trans Fatty Acids and Risk of Coronary Heart Disease Among Women," *Lancet* 341 (March 6, 1993): 581–585.

3. T. A. Mori and L. J. Beilin, "Omega-3 Fatty Acids and Inflammation," *Current Atherosclerosis Reports* 6, no. 6 (November 2004): 461–467; W. Elaine Hardman, "(n-3) Fatty Acids and Cancer Therapy," *The Journal of Nutrition* 134, suppl. 12 (December 2004): 3427S–3430S; A. A. Berbert et al., "Supplementation of Fish Oil and Olive Oil in Patients With Rheumatoid Arthritis," *Nutrition* 21, no. 2 (February 2005): 131–136; P. Guesnet et al., "Analysis of the 2nd Symposium: Anomalies of Fatty Acids, Ageing and Degenerating Pathologies," *Reproduction Nutrition Development* 44, no. 3 (May–June 2004): 263–271; J. A. Conquer et al., "Fatty Acid Analysis

of Blood Plasma of Patients With Alzheimer's D, Other Types of Dementia, and Cognitive Impairment," *Lipids* 35, no. 12 (December 2000): 1305–1312; L. A. Horrocks and Y. K. Yeo, "Health Benefits of Docosahexaenoic Acid (DHA)," *Pharmacological Research* 40, no. 3 (September 1999): 211–225; E. M. Hjerkinn et al., "Influence of Long-Term Intervention With Dietary Counseling, Long-Chain n-3 Fatty Acid Supplements, or Both on Circulating Markers of Endothelial Activation in Men With Long-Standing Hyperlipidemia," *Alternative Medicine Review* 81, no. 3 (March 2005): 583–589; and Joyce A. Nettleton and Robert Katz, "n-3 Long-Chain Polyunsaturated Fatty Acids in Type 2 Diabetes: A Review," *Journal of the American Dietetic Association* 105, no. 3 (March 2005): 428–440.

4. M. G. Enig, *Trans Fatty Acids in the Food Supply: A Comprehensive Report Covering 60 Years of Research*, 2nd edition (Silver Spring, MD: Enig Associates, Inc., 1995).

5. Don Colbert, *What Would Jesus Eat?* (Nashville: Thomas Nelson, 2001).

Chapter 12: Vitamin Confusion

1. "Multivitamin/mineral Supplements," National Institutes of Health Office of Dietary Supplements, accessed July 6, 2016, https://ods.od.nih.gov/factsheets/MVMS-HealthProfessional/.

2. "Heart Disease and Stroke Disease Statistics—At-a-Glance," American Heart Association and American Stroke Association, 2015 Heart Disease and Stroke Statistics Update, accessed July 6, 2016, http://www.heart.org/idc/groups/ahamah-public/@wcm/@sop/@smd/documents/downloadable/ucm_470704.pdf.

3. "Lifetime Risk of Developing or Dying From Cancer," American Cancer Society, accessed July 6, 2016, http://www.cancer.org/cancer/cancerbasics/lifetime-probability-of-developing-or-dying-from-cancer.

4. Balch, *Prescription for Nutritional Healing*, 13.

5. Ben Kim, "Synthetic vs. Natural Vitamins," Life Essentials Health Clinic, accessed July 6, 2016, http://chetday.com/naturalvitamin.htm.

6. "Hidden Hazards of Vitamin and Mineral Tablets," Life Essentials Health Clinic, accessed July 6, 2016, http://www.chetday.com/vitaminhazards.html.

7. Ibid.

8. Dominique Patton, "Oxidised Fish Oils on Market May Harm Consumer, Warns Researcher," NutraIngredients.com, October 20, 2005, accessed July 6, 2016, http://www.nutraingredients.com/news/ng.asp?id=63341-fish-oil-antioxidant.

9. Ibid.

10. Ibid.

Chapter 13: The Dangers of Mega-Dosing

1. Kim, "Hidden Hazards of Vitamin and Mineral Tablets."

2. "Peripheral Neuropathy and Vitamin B_6," University of Virginia Health System, accessed July 6, 2016, https://cancer.uvahealth.com/images-and-docs/neuropathy.pdf; "Vitamin B6: Fact Sheet for Consumers," National Institutes of Health, updated February 17, 2016, accessed July 6, 2016, https://ods.od.nih.gov/factsheets/VitaminB6-Consumer/.

3. "Dietary Supplement Fact Sheet: Vitamin A and Carotenoids," National Institutes of Health Office of Dietary Supplements.

4. Balch, *Prescription for Nutritional Healing,* 32.

5. Lonn et al., "Effects of Long-Term Vitamin E Supplementation on Cardiovascular Events and Cancer."

6. Patrick J. Skerrett, "High-Dose Vitamin C Linked to Kidney Stones in Men," Harvard Health Publications, Harvard Medical School, February 5, 2013, accessed August 23, 2016, http://www.health.harvard.edu/blog/high-dose-vitamin-c-linked-to-kidney-stones-in-men-201302055854.

7. "Vitamin D," National Institutes of Health Office of Dietary Supplements, accessed August 23, 2016, https://ods.od.nih.gov/factsheets/VitaminD-Consumer/.

8. Fletcher and Fairfield, "Vitamins for Chronic Disease Prevention in Adults."

9. "The Effect of Vitamin E and Beta Carotene on the Incidence of Lung Cancer and Other Cancers in Male Smokers," *New England Journal of Medicine.*

10. Ibid.

Chapter 14: How to Pick the Right Supplement

1. Paavo Airola, *How to Get Well* (Scottsdale, AZ: Health Plus Publishers, 1980), 210.

2. "Drugs and Supplements: Vitamin B_{12}," MayoClinic.com, accessed August 24, 2016, http://www.mayoclinic.com/print/vitamin-B12/Ns_patient-vitaminb12/METHOD=print.

Chapter 15: From ADD/ADHD to Thyroid Disorders

1. "Zinc: Fact Sheet for Health Professionals," National Institutes of Health, updated February 11, 2016, accessed July 6, 2016, https://ods.od.nih.gov/factsheets/Zinc-HealthProfessional/#en2.

2. "Vitamin C: Fact Sheet for Health Professionals," National Institutes of Health, updated February 11, 2016, accessed July 7, 2016, https://ods.od.nih.gov/factsheets/VitaminC-HealthProfessional/.

3. Ross Bloom, "92% of U.S. Population Have Vitamin Deficiency. Are You One of Them?" The Biostation, February 3, 2014, accessed July 8, 2016, http://thebiostation.com/resource-center/wellness/92-of-u-s-population-have-vitamin-deficiency-are-you-one-of-them/.

4. "L-Methylfoldate Dosage," Drugs.com, accessed October 20, 2016, https://www.drugs.com/dosage/l-matehyfolate.html.

5. Belinda Rowland and Teresa G. Odle, "Depression," Gale Encyclopedia of Alternative Medicine, 2005, accessed August 25, 2016, http://www.encyclopedia.com/utility/printdocument.aspx?id=1G2:3435100255.

6. T. C. Birdsall, "5-Hydroxytryptophan: A Clinically-Effective Serotonin Precursor," Alternative Medical Review 3, no. 4 (August 1998): 271–280, abstract viewed at PubMed.gov, accessed August 25, 2016, http://www.ncbi.nlm.nih.gov/pubmed/9727088.

7. "Mucuna Pruriens," Examine.com, accessed July 26, 2016, https://examine.com/supplements/mucuna-pruriens/; "4 Dopamine Boosters to Improve Depression Symptoms, Mood, and Motivation; UHN Daily, June 27, 2016, accessed July 26, 2016,

http://universityhealthnews.com/daily/depression/dopamine-supplements-for-improving-mood-and-motivation/.

8. "St. John's Wort and Depression: In Depth," National Center for Complementary and Integrative Health, updated September 2013, August 25, 2016, http://nccam.nih.gov/health/stjohnswort/sjw-and-depression.htm.

9. K. Lu, M. A. Gray, C. Oliver et al., "The Acute Effects of L-theanine in Comparison With Alprazolam on Anticipatory Anxiety in Humans," Hum Psychopharmacol 19, no. 7 (October 2004): 457–465, referenced in Tiesha D. Johnson, "Theanine vs. Xanax: Comparison of Effects," Life Extension Magazine, August 2007, accessed August 25, 2016, http://www.lef.org/magazine/mag2007/aug2007_report_stress_anxiety_02.htm.

10. "Turmeric," WebMD, accessed October 13, 2016, http://www.webmd.com/diet/supplement-guide-turmeric#1.

11. "Boswellia Serrata for Arthritis—Dosage & Research Review," Nootriment, accessed October 13, 2016, http://nootriment.com/boswellia-serrata-for-arthritis/.

12. Lane Lenard, Ward Dean, and Jim English, "Controlling Inflammation With Proteolytic Enzymes," Nutrition Review, April 24, 2013, accessed October 13, 2016, http://nutritionreview.org/2013/04/controlling-inflammation-proteolytic-enzymes/.

13. Jason Ramirez, "Krill Oil Optimizes Multimodal Arthritis Control," Life Extension Magazine, November 2011, accessed October 13, 2016, http://www.lifeextension.com/Magazine/2011/11/Krill-Oil-Optimizes-Multimodal-Arthritis-Control/Page-01.

14. Michael Downey, "Halt the Auto-Immune Attack of Arthritis," Life Extension Magazine, July 2012, accessed October 14, 2016, http://www.lifeextension.com/Magazine/2012/7/Hault-Auto-Immune-Attack-Of-Arthritis/Page-01.

15. Natural Standard Patient Monograph "Glucosamine," copyright 2016, Mayo Clinic, accessed October 14, 2016, http://www.mayoclinic.org/drugs-supplements/glucosamine/background/hrb-20059572.

16. "Glucosamine/Chondroitin Arthritis Intervention Trial (GAIT)," National Institutes of Health, accessed October 14, 2016, https://nccih.nih.gov/research/results/gait.

17. Mariko Oe et al., "Oral Hyaluronan Relieves Knee Pain: A Review," Nutrition Journal 15: (2015): 11, accessed October 14, 2016, doi: 10.1186/s12937-016-0128-2.

18. Lenard, Dean, and English, "Controlling Inflammation With Proteolytic Enzymes."

19. "Turmeric," WebMD.

20. Downey, "Halt the Auto-Immune Attack of Arthritis."

21. "Boswellia Serrata for Arthritis—Dosage & Research Review," Nootriment.

22. Mariko Oe et al., "Oral Hyaluronan Relieves Knee Pain: A Review."

23. Ramirez, "Krill Oil Optimizes Multimodal Arthritis Control."

24. I. Louw et al., "A Pilot Study of the Clinical Effects of a Mixture of Beta-Sisterol and Beta-Sisterol Glucoside in Active Rheumatoid Arthritis," *American Journal of Clinical Nutrition* 75 (2002): 351S (Abstract 40).

25. "Krill Oil is 'Safe, Well Tolerated and Effective,'" Mercola, February 2, 2010, accessed July 25, 2016, http://articles.mercola.com/sites/articles/archive/2010/02/02/krill-oil-is-safe-well-tolerated-and-effective.aspx.

26. Eugene Braunwald et al., *Harrison's Principles of Internal Medicine*, 15th edition (New York: McGraw-Hill, 2001).

27. Robert Iafelice, "Benefits of Wobenzym," updated May 6, 2015, accessed July 25, 2016, http://www.livestrong.com/article/161756-benefits-of-wobenzym/.

28. "Collagen Type II," WebMD, accessed July 25, 2016, http://www.webmd.com/vitamins-supplements/ingredientmono-714-collagen%20type%20ii.aspx?activeingredientid=714&activeingredientname=collagen%20type%20ii.

29. Alexis Black, "The Mineral Selenium Proves Itself as Powerful Anti-Cancer Medicine," NaturalNews.com, January 4, 2006, accessed August 26, 2016, http://www.naturalnews.com/016446_selenium_nutrition.html.

30. S. Y. Yu, B. L. Mao, P. Xiao et al., "Intervention Trial With Selenium for the Prevention of Lung Cancer Among Tin Miners in Yunnan, China. A Pilot Study," *Biological Trace Element Research* 24, no. 2 (February 1990): 105–108.

31. "Vitamin D for Cancer Prevention," MedicalNewsToday.com, February 7, 2007, accessed August 26, 2016, http://www.medicalnewstoday.com/articles/62413.php.

32. Suzan Clarke, "In Tests, Vitamin D Shrinks Breast Cancer Cells," ABCNews.com, February 22, 2010, accessed August 26, 2016, http://abcnews.go.com/print?id=9904415.

33. "Vitamin D for Cancer Prevention," MedicalNewsToday.com.

34. "How Curcumin Protects Against Cancer," Life Extension Magazine, March 2011, accessed July 25, 2016, http://www.lifeextension.com/magazine/2011/3/how-curcumin-protects-against-cancer/page-01.

35. Eileen M. Lynch, "Melatonin and Cancer Treatment," Life Extension, January 2004, accessed July 8, 2016, http://www.lifeextension.com/magazine/2004/1/report_melatonin/page-01.

36. Janet Renee, "Recommended Dosage of Pregnenolone," LiveStrong.com, updated February 19, 2014, accessed July 25, 2016, http://www.livestrong.com/article/503522-recommended-dosage-of-pregnenolone/.

37. D. C. Shungu, et al, "Increased Ventricular Lactate in Chronic Fatigue Syndrome. III. Relationships to Cortical Glutathione and Clinical Symptoms Implicate Oxidative Stress in Disorder Pathophysiology," *NMR Biomed* 25, no. 9 (September 2012): 1073–1087.

38. P. C. Tullson and R. L. Terjung, "Adenine Nucleotide Synthesis in Exercising and Endurance-Trained Skeletal Muscle," *American Journal of Physiology* 261, no. 2 (C342–C347), referenced in Julius G. Goepp, "Rejuvenate Cardiac Cellular Energy Production," LifeExtensionVitamins.com, May 2008, accessed August 28, 2016, http://www.lifeextensionvitamins.com/may08denyohe.html.

39. "Royal Jelly," WebMD, accessed July 11, 2016, http://www.webmd.com/vitamins-supplements/ingredientmono-503-ROYAL+JELLY.aspx?activeIngredientId=503&activeIngredientName=ROYAL+JELLY&source=0.

40. Linus Pauling, *Vitamin C and the Common Cold* (San Francisco: W. H. Freeman, 1970).

41. Linus Pauling, "The Significance of the Evidence of Ascorbic Acid and the Common Cold," *Proceedings of the National Academy of Sciences of the USA* 68 (November 1971): 2678–2681.

42. Jennifer Warner, "Low Vitamin D Levels Linked to Colds," WebMD, February 23, 2009, http://www.webmd.com/cold-and-flu/news/20090223/low-vitamin-d-levels-linked-to-colds.

43. Sherif B. Mossad et al., "Zinc Gluconate Lozenges for Treating the Common Cold," Annals of Internal Medicine 125 (July 15, 1996): 81–88, accessed August 28, 2016, http://www.annals.org/cgi/content/abstract/125/2/.

44. Lynda Liu, "Fighting the Flu With Alternative Remedies," January 7, 2000, accessed August 28, 2016, http://www.rense.com/politics6/flufight.htm.

45. Ibid.

46. Ibid.

47. R. T. Mathie, J Frye, and P Fisher, "Homeopathic Oscillococcinum for Preventing and Treating Influenza and Influenza-Like Illness," Cochrane Database System Review 1 (January 28, 2015), accessed July 11, 2016, http://www.ncbi.nlm.nih.gov/pubmed/25629583.

48. Gordon Pedersen, *A Fighting Chance: How to Win the War Against Bacteria, Viruses & Mold With Silver,* 2nd ed. (n.p.: Sound Concepts, 2008), 19–20.

49. "Vitamin D Is the 'It' Nutrient of the Moment," ScienceDaily.com, January 14, 2009, accessed July 12, 2016, http://www.sciencedaily.com/releases/2009/01/090112121821.htm.

50. Recommended Dietary Allowances, 10th edition (Washington, DC: National Academy Press, 1989); "Chromium," National Institutes of Health, accessed August 28, 2016, https://ods.od.nih.gov/factsheets/%20chromium-HealthProfessional/.

51. Neal D. Barnard, *Dr. Neal Barnard's Program for Reversing Diabetes* (New York: Rodale, 2007), 142.

52. Ibid., 143.

53. Richard A. Anderson, "Chromium in the Prevention and Control of Diabetes," *Diabetes and Metabolism* 26, no. 1 (2000): 22–27, as cited in Frank Murray, *Natural Supplements for Diabetes* (Laguna Beach, CA: Basic Health Publications, Inc. 2007), 114.

54. Ibid.

55. Richard A. Anderson, "Chromium, Glucose Intolerance and Diabetes," *Journal of the American College of Nutrition* 17, no. 6 (1998): 548–555.

56. Mark A. Mitchell, "Lipoic Acid: A Multitude of Metabolic Health Benefits," Life Extension magazine, October 2007, accessed August 28, 2016, http://www.lef.org/LEFCMS/aspx/PrintVersionMagic.aspx?CmsID=115115.

57. "How Does Fiber Affect Blood Glucose Levels?," Joslin Diabetes Center, accessed August 28, 2016, http://www.joslin.org/managing_your_diabetes_697.asp.

58. James W. Anderson, *Dr. Anderson's High-Fiber Fitness Plan* (Lexington, KY: University Press of Kentucky, 1994), 14.

59. Michael Murray, "What Makes People Fat, Why Diets Don't Work, and What Triggers Appetite?," Life Extension Vitamins, accessed August 28, 2016, http://www.lifeextensionvitamins.com/whmapefawhyd.html.

60. "Good Bye to Fad Diets, Revolutionary Natural Fibre Discovered in Canada," MedicalNewsToday.com, August 14, 2004, accessed August 28, 2016, http://www.medicalnewstoday.com/articles/12058.php.

61. Alam Khan et al., "Cinnamon Improves Glucose and Lipids of People With Type 2 Diabetes," December 2003, 26 no. 12 (December 2003): 3215–3218, accessed July 13, 2016, http://care.diabetesjournals.org/content/26/12/3215.

62. Andrea Markowitz, "Forbidden Fruits and Other Foods," *Chicago Tribune*, July 26, 2010, accessed July 7, 2016, http://articles.chicagotribune.com/2010-07-26/health/sc-health-0723-allergies-food-20100723_1_food-intolerance-food-allergies-anaphylactic-reaction.

63. "Bacteria That Protect Against Food Allergies Identified," FARS News Agency, August 29, 2014, accessed July 25, 2016, http://www.lifeextension.com/news/lefdailynews?NewsID=22793&Section=NUTRITION.

64. D. Frances, "Feverfew for Acute Headaches: Does It Work?" *Medical Herbalism: A Clinical Newsletter for the Clinical Practitioner* 7 no. 4 (Winter 1995–1996), 1–2.

65. C. Boehnke et al., "High-Dose Riboflavin Treatment Is Efficacious In Migraine Prophylaxis: An Open Study in a Tertiary Care Centre," *European Journal of Neurology* 11, no. 7 (2004): 475–477, abstract viewed at PubMed.gov, accessed October 20, 2016, https://www.ncbi.nlm.nih.gov/pubmed/15257686.

66. Darrell Hulisz "Does Butterbur Prevent Migraines?," February 2, 2015, accessed October 20, 2016, http://www.medscape.com/viewarticle/838939.

67. Perry Marcone, "Generate Fresh Mitochondria With PQQ," Life Extension Magazine, February 2011, accessed July 25, 2016, http://www.lifeextension.com/magazine/2011/2/Generate-Fresh-Mitochondria-with-PQQ/Page-01.

68. Alexander Leaf, "On the Reanalysis of the GISSI-Prevenzione," *Circulation* 105, no. 16 (2002): 1874–1875.

69. Christine M. Albert et al., "Blood Levels of Long-Chain n-3 Fatty Acids and the Risk of Sudden Death," *New England Journal of Medicine* 346, no. 15 (April 11, 2002): 1113–1118.

70. Kimmi Le, "Nutritional Dangers of Acid Reflux Medications," *Life Extension Magazine*, June 2013, accessed July 26, 2016, http://www.lifeextension.com/magazine/2013/6/nutritional-dangers-of-acid-reflux-medications/page-01; "Gastroesophageal Reflux Disease (GERD)," Life Extension, accessed July 26, 2016, http://www.lifeextension.com/Protocols/Gastrointestinal/Gastroesophageal-Reflux/Page-08.

71. Laura Cox, "How to Get Rid of Acid Reflux? Try D-Limonene," RefluxMD, accessed July 26, 2016, http://www.refluxmd.com/how-to-get-rid-of-acid-reflux/.

72. Russell Martin, "Natural Relief From Heartburn!," Life Extension Magazine, September 2006, accessed July 26, 2016, http://www.lifeextension.com/magazine/2006/9/cover_heartburn/page-01.

73. "Mastic," WebMD, accessed August 28, 2016, http://www.webmd.com/vitamins-supplements/ingredientmono-565-mastic.aspx?activeingredientid=565.

74. Lester Packer, *The Antioxidant Miracle* (New York: John Wiley and Sons, Inc., 1999).

75. Stephanie Watson, "Can Hepatitis C Be Cured?," reviewed May 20, 2016, accessed July 26, 2016, http://www.webmd.com/hepatitis/features/cure?page=3.

76. L. Brown et al., "Cholesterol-Lowering Effects of Dietary Fiber: A Meta-Analysis," *American Journal of Clinical Nutrition* 69, no. 1 (January 1999).

77. Joseph Mercola, *The No-Grain Diet* (New York: E. P. Dutton, 2003).

78. J. G. Coniglio, "How Does Fish Oil Lower Plasma Triglycerides?" *Nutrition Reviews* 50 (July 1992): 195–197.

79. "Fish: What Pregnant Women and Parents Should Know," FDA, June 2014, accessed July 26, 2016, http://www.fda.gov/Food/FoodborneIllnessContaminants/Metals/ucm393070.htm.

80. Michael Downey, "Olive Leaf Safely Modulates Blood Pressure," Life Extension Magazine, March 2012, accessed August 29, 2016, https://www.lef.org/magazine/mag2012/mar2012_Olive-Leaf-Safely-Modulates-Blood-Pressure_01.htm.

81. Nadia Arumugam, "Drinking Beetroot Juice Every Day Can Help Lower Blood Pressure by 7 Percent," Forbes, April 25, 2013, accessed August 29, 2016, http://www.forbes.com/sites/nadiaarumugam/2013/04/25/drinking-beetroot-juice-every-day-can-help-lower-blood-pressure-by-7-percent/.

82. A. Herrera-Arellano et al., "Effectiveness and Tolerability of a Standardized Extract From Hibiscus Sabdariffa in Patients With Mild to Moderate Hypertension, A Controlled and Randomized Clinical Trial," *Phytomedicine* 11, no. 5 (July 2004): 375–382.

83. "Celery," WebMD, accessed July 18, 2016, http://www.webmd.com/vitamins-supplements/ingredientmono-882-celery.aspx?activeingredientid=882&activeingredientname=celery.

84. F. C. Luft and M. H. Weinberger, "Sodium Intake and Essential Hypertension," *Hypertension* 4, no. 5 (September–October 1982): 14–19.

85. M. Sabater-Molina et al., "Dietary Fructooligosaccharides and Potential Benefits on Health," *Journal of Physiology and Biochemistry* 65, no. 3 (September 2009).

86. Lester Packer, *The Antioxidant Miracle* (New York: John Wiley and Sons Inc., 1999).

87. "Alzheimer's and Vitamin E," *New England Journal of Medicine* (April 1997).

88. Steven Bratman and David Kroll, *Natural Health Bible* (n.p.: Prima Health, 1999).

89. Alan Smithee, "Feed Your Brain!," January 2011, accessed October 20, 2016, www.lifeextension.com/magazine/2011/1/feed-your-brain/page-01.

90. T. P. Ng et al., "Curry Consumption and Cognitive Function in the Elderly," American Journal of Epidemiology, 165, no. 9 (November 1, 2006): 898–906, abstract viewed at PubMed.gov, accessed October 20, 2016, https://www.ncbi.nlm.nih.gov/pubmed/16870699.

91. "Super Food: Let's Talk Turmeric," Alzheimers.net, August 4, 2014, accessed October 20, 2016, http://www.alzheimers.net/2013-07-29/turmeric-and-alzheimers/.

92. Perry Marcone, Generate Fresh Mitochondria With PQQ," LifeExtension, February 2011, accessed October 20, 2016, http://www.lifeextension.com/magazine/2011/2/Generate-Fresh-Mitochondria-with-PQQ/Page-01.

93. "Estrovera," Metagenics, accessed July 26, 2016, http://www.metagenics.com/estrovera.

94. "Rhubarb May Cool Hot Flashes," WebMD, September 15, 2006, accessed July 26, 2016, http://www.webmd.com/menopause/news/20060915/rhubarb-may-cool-hot-flashes.

95. "Flaxseed," Life Extension Magazine, October 2008, accessed July 26, 2016, http://www.lifeextension.com/magazine/2008/10/flaxseed/page-01.

96. "Green Coffee Bean Extract," *Life Extension Magazine*, February 2012.

97. "Iodine Deficiency," American Thyroid Association, June 4, 2012, accessed August 29, 2016, http://www.thyroid.org/iodine-deficiency/.

98. "Mucuna Pruriens," Examine.com.

99. Francine Juhasz, "Symptoms of Dopamine Deficiency," Livestrong.com, April 14, 2015, accessed July 26, 2016, http://www.livestrong.com/article/346030-symptoms-of-dopamine-deficiency/.

100. J. A. Marlett, M. I. McBurney, J. L. Slavin, and American Dietetic Association, "Position of the American Dietetic Association: Health Implications of Dietary Fiber," *Journal of the American Dietetic Association* 102, no. 7 (2002): 993–1000.

101. N. C. Howarth, E. Saltzman, and S. B. Roberts, "Dietary Fiber and Weight Regulation," *Nutrition Review* 59, no. 5 (2001): 129–138.

102. Andrew Weil, "7-Keto: Supplement to Speed Metabolism?," DrWeil.com, accessed August 29, 2016, http://www.drweil.com/drw/u/QAA401158/7Keto-Supplement-to-Speed-Metabolism.html.

103. "7-Keto-DHEA," WebMD.com, accessed August 29, 2016, http://www.webmd.com/vitamins-supplements/ingredientmono-835-7-KETO-DHEA.aspx?activeIngredientId=835&activeIngredientName=7-KETO-DHEA.

104. Weil, "7-Keto: Supplement to Speed Metabolism?"

105. J. L. Zenk, J. L. Frestedt, and M. A. Kuskowski, "HUM5007, a Novel Combination of Thermogenic Compounds, and 3-Acetyl-7-Oxo-Dehydroepiandrosterone: Each Increases the Resting Metabolic Rate of Overweight Adults," Journal of Nutritional Biochemistry 18, no. 9 (September 2007): 629–634; Michael Davidson et al., "Safety and Pharmacokinetic Study With Escalating Doses of 3-Acetyl-7-Oxo-Dehydroepiandrosterone in Healthy Male Volunteers," *Clinical Investigative Medicine* 23, no. 5 (October 2000): 300–310, abstract accessed August 29, 2016, http://www.ncbi.nlm.nih.gov/pubmed/11055323.

106. Rekha Mankad, "Heart Attack," February 11, 2016, accessed July 22, 2016, http://www.mayoclinic.org/diseases-conditions/heart-attack/expert-answers/calcium-supplements/faq-20058352.

107. William Davis, "Protecting Bone and Arterial Health With Vitamin K_2," Life Extension Magazine, March 2008, accessed July 25, 2016, http://www.lifeextension.com/magazine/2008/3/protecting-bone-and-arterial-health-with-vitamin-k2/Page-01.

108. D. Feskanich et al., "Vitamin A Intake and Hip Fractures Among Postmenopausal Women," abstract, Journal of American Medical Association 287, no. 1 (January 2002): 47–54, accessed August 29, 2016, http://www.ncbi.nlm.nih.gov/pubmed/11754708.

109. "How to Best Absorb Calcium Supplements," eHow.com, accessed August 29, 2016, http://www.ehow.com/how_3953_absorb-calcium-supplements.html.

110. "Magnesium in Depth," BodyAndFitness.com, accessed July 6, 2009, http://www.bodyandfitness.com/Information/Health/Research/magnesium.htm.

111. M. Kaneki et al., "Japanese Fermented Soybean Food as the Major Determinant of the Large Geographic Difference in Circulating Levels of Vitamin K_2: Possible Implications for Hip-fracture Risk," Nutrition 17, no. 4 (2001): 315–321, as quoted in William Davis, "Protecting Bone and Arterial Health With Vitamin K2,"

Life Extension Magazine, March 2008, accessed August 29, 2016, http://www.lef.org/magazine
/mag2008/mar2008_Protecting-Bone-And-Arterial-Health-With-Vitamin-K2_01.htm.

112. Steven M. Plaza and Davis W. Lamson, "Vitamin K_2 in Bone Metabolism and Osteoporosis," *Alternative Medicine Review* 10, no. 1 (2005): 24–35, accessed August 29, 2016, http://www.altmedrev.com/publications/10/1/24.pdf; H Asakura et al., "Vitamin K Administration to Elderly Patients With Osteoporosis Induces No Hemostatic Activation, Even in Those With Suspected Vitamin K Deficiency," Osteoporos Int 12 (2001): 996–1000.

113. Joseph Pizzorno, "Strong Bones for Life—Naturally (Part 2)," WebMD blog, October 16, 2008, accessed August 29, 2016, http://blogs.webmd.com/integrative-medicine-wellness/2008/10/strong-bones-for-life-naturally-part-2.html.

114. Ward Dean, "Strontium: Breakthrough Against Osteoporosis," American Academy of Anti-Aging Medicine, May 5, 2004, accessed July 19, 2016, http://www.worldhealth.net/news/strontium_breakthrough_against_osteoporo.

115. P. J. Meunier et al., "The Effects of Strontium Ranelate on the Risk of Vertebral Fracture in Women With Postmenopausal Osteoporosis," New England Journal of Medicine 350, no. 5 (January 2004): 459–468, accessed July 19, 2016, http://content.nejm.org/cgi/content/abstract/350/5/459.

116. Dean, "Strontium: Breakthrough Against Osteoporosis."

117. "Premenstrual Syndrome," Life Extension, accessed July 26, 2016, http://www.lifeextension.com/protocols/female-reproductive/premenstrual-syndrome/page-06?p=1.

118. "How Curcumin Protects Against Cancer," *Life Extension Magazine*.

119. Stephen Strum and William Faloon, "Beta-Sitosterol," Life Extension Magazine, June 2005, accessed July 25, 2016, http://www.lifeextension.com/magazine/2005/6/report_prostate/Page-01; "Beta-Sitosterol," WebMD, accessed July 25, 2016, http://www.webmd.com/vitamins-supplements/ingredientmono-939-beta-sitosterol.aspx?activeingredientid=939&activeingredientname=beta-sitosterol.

120. John Boudreau, "'King's Herb' One of Many From Vietnam Taking Hold in U.S. Market," Mercury News, June 26, 2012, accessed August 4, 2016, http://www.mercurynews.com/ci_20942411/kings-herb-one-many-from-vietnam-taking-hold; "Research," Crila Health, accessed August 4, 2016, https://crilahealth.com/prostate-uterine-menopause-research?mnu=6.

121. "Astaxanthin: The Antioxidant That Makes Fish Oil Work Better," Mercola; "Astaxanthin," WebMD.

122. John O. A. Pagano. *Healing Psoriasis* (Englewood Cliffs, NJ: The Pagano Organization Inc, 2000).

123. M. Nazzaro-Porro, "Azelaic Acid," *Journal of the American Academy of Dermatology* 17 (1987): 1033–1041.

124. I. V. Zhdanova et al., "Sleep-inducing Effects of Low Doses of Melatonin Ingested in the Evening," Clinical Pharmacology and Therapeutics 57, no. 5 (May 1995): 552–558, abstract accessed August 29, 2016, http://www.ncbi.nlm.nih.gov/pubmed/7768078.

125. "Rapid Anxiety and Stress Relief," Discover Nutrition, accessed August 29, 2016, http://www.discovernutrition.com/l-theanine.html.

126. A. Fidanza, "Therapeutic Action of Pantothenic Acid," *International Journal for Vitamin and Nutrition Research* 24, supplement (1983): 53–67.

127. Nancy Piccone, "The Silent Epidemic of Iodine Deficiency," Life Extension Magazine, October 2011, accessed July 26, 2016, http://www.lifeextension.com/magazine/2011/10/the-silent-epidemic-of-iodine-deficiency/Page-01.

128. Sage Kalmus, "Herbs That Help in T4 to T3 Conversion," August 16, 2013, accessed July 26, 2016, http://www.livestrong.com/article/498835-herbs-that-help-in-t4-to-t3-conversion/.

INDEX

Symbols

A

C

N

O

P

T

U

V

W

X

Y

Z